PULMONARY REHABILITATION

PULMONARY REHABILITATION

AK Simonds
*Consultant in Respiratory Medicine, Royal Brompton Hospital,
London, United Kingdom*

J-F Muir
*Professor of Respiratory Medicine, Service de Pneumologie, CHU de
Rouen, Hôpital de Bois-Guillaume, Rouen, France*

DJ Pierson
*Professor of Medicine, Division of Pulmonary and Critical Care
Medicine, University of Washington, Seattle, Washington, USA*

BMJ
Publishing
Group

© BMJ Publishing Group 1996

First published in 1996
by the BMJ Publishing Group, BMA House, Tavistock Square,
London WC1H 9JR

British Library Cataloguing in Publication Data

A catalogue record for this book is available
from the British Library

ISBN 0-7279-1022-1

Typeset, printed and bound in Great Britain by
Latimer Trend & Company Ltd, Plymouth

Contents

Contributors

Michael J Belman
Pulmonary Physiology Laboratory, Cedars-Sinai Medical Center, Los Angeles, California, USA

CJ Clarke
Hairmyres Hospital, East Kilbride, Glasgow, UK

Trevor Clay (deceased)
Former General Secretary of the Royal College of Nursing and Founder/President of Breathe Easy Club, British Lung Foundation, London, UK

J Randall Curtis
Assistant Professor, Department of Medicine, University of Washington, Seattle, Washington, USA

Richard A Deyo
Professor, Departments of Medicine and Health Services, University of Washington, Seattle, Washington, USA

PR Edwards
Department of Medicine and Pharmacology, University of Sheffield, Royal Hallamshire Hospital, Sheffield, UK

Roger S Goldstein
Director, Program in Respiratory Rehabilitation, Division of Respiratory Medicine, Department of Medicine, University of Toronto, Ontario, Canada

P Howard
Department of Medicine and Pharmacology, University of Sheffield, Royal Hallamshire Hospital, Sheffield, UK

Leonard D Hudson
Professor, Department of Medicine, University of Washington, Seattle, Washington, USA

John Isitt
National Organiser, Breathe Easy Club, British Lung Foundation, London, UK

J-F Muir
Service de Pneumologie, CHU de Rouen, Hôpital de
Bois-Guillaume, France

Michael G Pearson
Consultant Physician, Aintree Chest Centre, Liverpool, UK

Thomas L Petty
Professor of Medicine, HealthOne Center for Health Sciences
Education, Denver, Colorado, USA

Jennifer A Pryor
Head of Physiotherapy, Royal Brompton Hospital, London, UK

AK Simonds
Consultant in Respiratory Medicine, Royal Brompton Hospital,
London, UK

F Smeets
Centre Hospitalier de Sainte-Ode, Belgium

MI Walters
Department of Medicine and Pharmacology, University of
Sheffield, Royal Hallamshire Hospital, Sheffield, UK

JC Waterhouse
Chief Technician, Department of Medicine and Pharmacology,
University of Sheffield, Royal Hallamshire Hospital, Sheffield,
UK

Barbara A Webber
Formerly Head of Physiotherapy, Royal Brompton Hospital,
London, UK

H Worth
Professor and Chairman, Medical Department 1, Fuerth
Hospital, Fuerth, Germany

Preface

In 1974 a special committee of the American College of Chest Physicians proposed the following definition of rehabilitation in patients with respiratory disorders, primarily individuals with chronic obstructive pulmonary disease (COPD):

> Pulmonary rehabilitation is: An art of medical practice wherein an individually tailored multidisciplinary program is formulated which, through accurate diagnosis, therapy, emotional support and education, stabilizes or reverses both the physio- and psychopathology of pulmonary diseases and attempts to return the patient to the highest possible functional capacity allowed by his pulmonary handicap and overall life situation.

Initial enthusiasm during the federally funded studies in the United States of America in the 1960s and early 1970s was followed by a decade in which pulmonary rehabilitation enjoyed less favour. This was in part because few means were at hand to study much of its multidisciplinary content in an objective manner. Research focused mainly on physiological outcomes such as exercise capacity, which tended to show little improvement in most patients, rather than using quality of life as an evaluation tool.

In 1986 a provocative paper by Make[1] pointed out that it was in fact possible, after everything had been done to maximise lung function with pharmaceutical agents and other conventional medical techniques, to bring about further improvement in the functional level of patients with severe COPD by pulmonary rehabilitation. In his paper Make emphasised the importance of both diagnostic and therapeutic modalities in improving quality of life, including both psychological and educational aspects. During the past 20 years a considerable amount of work has been done in three important areas of pulmonary rehabilitation in COPD: improvement in the degree of airflow obstruction; prevention and treatment of complications; and assessment of improvement in the quality of life. The myth of the 1970s is truly becoming the reality of the 1990s, as the reader will see in this book. However, there is much to be done. An NIH workshop in pulmonary rehabilitation research in 1993[2] highlighted the issues that still need addressing:

- What are the long term benefits?
- What are the roles of the various components of rehabilitation schemes (exercise, ventilatory muscle training, dyspnoea management, etc.)?
- What is the effect of pulmonary rehabilitation in respiratory disorders other than COPD?

To emphasise a more evaluative approach a new definition was proposed which stresses the pluralistic nature of the enterprise, but deliberately avoids labelling pulmonary rehabilitation as an "art":

> Pulmonary rehabilitation is a multidimensional continuum of services directed to persons with pulmonary disease and their families, usually by an interdisciplinary team of specialists, with the goal of achieving and maintaining the individual's maximal level of independence and functioning in the community.

To open this book Petty traces the development of the large US pulmonary rehabilitation schemes and discusses the practical application of what has been learned in those programmes in the contemporary community hospital and private practice settings. Exercise reconditioning is at the heart of pulmonary rehabilitation and two reviews cover aspects of this important component. Belman discusses the overall concept of exercise reconditioning and reviews the efficacy of various approaches, including upper body exercise. Goldstein then examines the more specialised area of techniques aimed specifically at training the ventilatory muscles, placing the rationale for such training in the context of available experimental data.

The critical role of pharmacological interventions in early and late stage COPD, and smoking cessation, are analysed in subsequent chapters. Physical therapies have long been employed in the management of COPD, not all of them based on firm evidence. Pryor and Webber consider the contribution of physiotherapy techniques to pulmonary rehabilitation schemes in chapter 6.

For many patients effective pulmonary rehabilitation involves the use of technology as well as techniques. Foremost in this respect is long term oxygen therapy, the rationale, efficacy, and practical application of which are reviewed by the Sheffield group. Next, Muir addresses the rapidly expanding field of mechanical ventilatory assistance using less invasive techniques for long term support and also for short term care during acute exacerbations, including the use of nasal mask ventilation in intermediate respiratory care units and other innovative approaches.

As the results of all these interventions must focus not only on physiological improvement and prolongation of life, but also on improvement in the well being of the patient, the book continues with a chapter on quality of life assessment in those with chronic pulmonary insufficiency. In this overview, Curtis, Deyo, and Hudson discuss the techniques that are available for quantifying the components that comprise "quality of life", and review how these indispensable tools can be used most effectively, both by clinicians managing individual patients with disabling pulmonary disease and in future studies.

The practical aspects of setting up a pulmonary rehabilitation scheme, and the outcome of such schemes in individuals with pulmonary disease other than COPD, are discussed in chapters 10 and 11. The topic of travel for patients with chronic pulmonary disease, which relies heavily on the appropriate use of technological support and sensible planning, is reviewed by Smeets.

Finally, the perspective of the individual with respiratory disease should be acknowledged by all those responsible for developing rehabilitation schemes. We are grateful to the late Trevor Clay for swapping hats to provide a consumers' view of respiratory health care.

Chapters 2, 3, 7, 9, 10, 12, and 13 all originally appeared in the review series in *Thorax* devoted to pulmonary rehabilitation, edited by J-F Muir and DJ Pierson, and have only been changed slightly for publication in this volume.

AK Simonds, J-F Muir, and
DJ Pierson
January 1996

1 Make BJ. Pulmonary rehabilitation: myth or reality? *Clin Chest Med* 1986;7: 519–40.
2 Fisher AP. NIH Workshop Summary. Pulmonary rehabilitation research. *Am J Respir Crit Care Med* 1994;**149**:825–33.

1 Pulmonary rehabilitation: present status and future directions—an overview*

THOMAS L PETTY

Pulmonary rehabilitation as a process

Pulmonary rehabilitation is not a single form of therapy, but rather a systematic and often personally oriented approach to comprehensive treatment for patients with advanced impairment and disability, primarily from chronic obstructive pulmonary disease (COPD).[1] The techniques and approaches to pulmonary rehabilitation are, however, applicable to other chronic respiratory disease states such as those associated with interstitial pneumonitis/fibrosis, cystic fibrosis, thoracic deformities, and less common disorders. In brief, pulmonary rehabilitation should be considered as a form of advanced integrative care which goes beyond "ordinary care".

Essential components of a pulmonary rehabilitation programme

Pulmonary rehabilitation is appropriately considered, comprehensive care for patients with chronic respiratory disorders. The salient features of pulmonary rehabilitation are considered below.

* Based in part on a presentation made to the Annual General Meeting of the Hong Kong Thoracic Society and Hong Kong Chapter of the American College of Chest Physicians, 22 April 1993.

1

Patient and family education

Education is important in all chronic disease states. Both the patient and the family should understand the objectives, methodologies, and realistic goals of care. Patient education can be individually taught, but is most commonly offered in small group sessions. Education includes a review of the disease states, anatomy and physiology of the lung, and pharmacological therapies employed, and the rationale behind the various techniques of breathing re-training and exercise is demonstrated. When appropriate, the techniques of home oxygen therapy are taught, and pamphlets and short books are used to supplement these personal instructions.[2]

Pharmacological agents

Bronchoactive drugs

The inhaled β agonists are the most widely used agents to help patients reduce dyspnoea through bronchodilatation, even in advanced stages of COPD. A substantial number of, indeed most, patients with COPD have some measurable improvement in forced expiratory volume in 1 second (FEV$_1$, flow), forced vital capacity (FVC, volume), or sometimes both.[3] Many patients use β agonists throughout the day, that is, whenever they face troublesome dyspnoea. This may occur as frequently as every 1–2 hours, which is the duration of the peak effect of the commonly available inhaled β agonists delivered by metered dose inhalers (MDIs). In general, oral β agonists are reserved for those patients who will not or cannot use an MDI properly. Oral β agonists are no more effective than inhaled agents and, in fact, are less effective in providing immediate improvement. The major side effects of tremor and tachycardia limit their usefulness.

Anticholinergics generally produce a greater and longer period of sustained bronchodilatation than the β agonists.[4] Ipratropium bromide (Atrovent), the only anticholinergic available in the United States of America in a metered dose inhaler, has become a cornerstone agent. Other anticholinergics such as oxitropium are available in Europe and elsewhere. Inhaled anticholinergics do not produce tremor and, as they are poorly absorbed, have few side effects. Urinary retention, glaucoma, and the drying of bronchial secretions generally do not occur with these agents. Caution should be exercised in patients with glaucoma. A spacer is helpful in

2

avoiding spraying the product into the eyes, which would be harmful in these patients.

Until recently the theophyllines were the most widely used bronchodilators in the United States of America. Theophyllines are relatively weak bronchodilators compared with either the inhaled β agonists or anticholinergics. Although theophyllines were shown in controlled clinical trials to provide slight improvements in airflow and volume, as well as an improvement in blood gases, the magnitude of these changes is modest.[5] It is likely that the benefit achieved in most patients is due to the extrabronchial activities of theophylline, such as improving respiratory muscle function.

Corticosteroids are also widely used with various strategies in COPD. Corticosteroids are most commonly used to help deal with exacerbations of disease that result in acute respiratory insufficiency. One controlled clinical trial showed that cortico-steroids could improve ventilatory function to a statistically significant degree but the clinical impact was small.[6] Whether or not corticosteroids can forestall the progress of moderate or severe COPD has been the subject of extensive observations,[7 8] but thus far no controlled clinical trials have been completed. Most experts in the field believe that corticosteroids can favour-ably modify the course taken by some patients with COPD. Corticosteroids have also been shown to identify some patients with an unexpected reversible component to their disease. This is true even in advanced cases, including patients who require long term home oxygen therapy.[9]

Mucoactive drugs are widely used in Europe, but until recently have been used sparsely in North America.[10] One extensive controlled clinical trial showed a marked reduction in cough severity, cough frequency, chest tightness, and dyspnoea, and an improved global feeling of well being for many patients with moderate COPD.[11] Most pulmonary physicians consider iodinated glycerol, the only adequately studied drug in this class, to be adjunctive therapy and not a replacement for any other drugs in the so called bronchoactive class. However, iodinated glycerol is no longer available in the United States of America. Pharmacological therapies are considered in detail in Chapter 4.

Strategic drugs

At the top of the list of strategic drugs come the antibiotics. Although many patients with COPD have exacerbations of cough, dyspnoea, increased and coloured sputum, and bacterial pathogens in the sputum, the exact role of bacterial pathogens in these exacerbations remains unclear. It is most likely that virus infections are the inciting cause of the exacerbations, with bacterial invasion occurring secondarily. One well designed, controlled, clinical trial demonstrated clinical effectiveness with the use of antimicrobial agents in some, but not all, patients with exacerbations of chronic bronchitis.[12] An alternative theory is that these exacerbations of COPD result from non-microbial inflammatory processes. This may well be the reason why corticosteroids are so valuable in exacerbations of disease.

Nicotine replacement must, of course, be considered in all patients who are still smoking as they enter a pulmonary rehabilitation programme. Hopefully, most patients requiring pulmonary rehabilitation have long since decided to abstain from the product that caused the disease process in the first place. A discussion of all the strategies of nicotine replacement is given in chapter 5. Beyond a doubt, the patient's commitment to quit, the assistance of a physician or other health workers in helping the patient to alter behaviour patterns that sustain the smoking habit or addiction, and nicotine replacement to deal with withdrawal symptoms all offer an effective strategy in smoking cessation. Nicotine polacrilex (Nicorette) and four different preparations of transdermal nicotine (Habitrol, Nicoderm, cinotrol, and Prostep) are now available in the United States of America. In the United Kingdom, the preparations available are Nicorette, Nicotinell, and Nicoril. Controlled clinical trials have indicated considerable success when transdermal nicotine replacement is added to behavioural modification.[13]

Influenza virus vaccine is advised each autumn to deal with real or potential epidemics of an infection that often devastates patients with moderate to severe forms of chronic respiratory insufficiency. A polyvalent vaccine is prepared from the expected strains, based upon worldwide epidemiological considerations. In general, a single injection of the polyvalent vaccine is given each October or November to all patients with any degree of respiratory insufficiency and should be given to everyone over the age of 50.[14] Pneumococcal vaccine should be offered once in a lifetime and perhaps as often as every five years to help reduce the risk of complications from this common bacterial pathogen.[15] Amantadine may be an effective oral preventive against influenza A strains for patients who will not

4

or cannot take the vaccine, when there has been insufficient time to immunise in the face of an epidemic, or in patients who are institutionalised along with others who have influenza.

Breathing exercises and re-training

A great deal of study has been made into the techniques of breathing training, strengthening the breathing muscles, and coordinating the breathing process. More studies of pursed lip breathing have been reported than other controlled breathing techniques. Pursed lip breathing slows respiration and increases the depth of each breath; it also helps to improve oxygen transfer across the lungs,[16 17] and relieves dyspnoea during exercise. Various techniques of breathing exercises have been employed. These can include maximum voluntary ventilation manoeuvres, the use of progressive resistive inspiratory devices, including both flow and threshold resistors, and other techniques (see chapter 3).[18 19]

Systemic exercise

It has been known for a long time that patients can learn to walk greater distances with less dyspnoea and at a lower heart and respiratory rate through exercise training (see chapter 2).[20 21] The mechanisms behind these improvements are complex. Part of the physiological benefits of systemic exercising includes a reduction in exercise related lactic acidosis, probably in part via improved cardiovascular responses.[22] The exercise tolerance of many patients with advanced COPD is, however, limited by intolerable dyspnoea. Some people with milder forms of the disease have cardiovascular limitations or are limited by the mechanics of breathing and generalised muscle weakness. Impaired pulmonary mechanics and a heightened sense of dyspnoea are the greatest limiting factors in most patients with moderate to severe COPD. Patients can be trained to tolerate dyspnoea through a variety of exercise techniques. Normal walking on the level and out of doors, with increasing times and distances, is a simple approach that can be used by almost all ambulatory patients.

Oxygen

Oxygen is the only therapy that is often employed both with and without the other techniques of pulmonary rehabilitation; it has been shown to alter favourably the outcome in chronic stable patients who have hypoxaemia associated with advanced stages of

COPD.[23][24] Two major multicentre trials, when taken together, indicate that, without oxygen, survival for those who have chronic stable hypoxaemia with advanced COPD is poor. Survival is improved with oxygen given for 12–15 hours per day, including the hours of sleep, from stationary sources. Survival is best, however, when oxygen is given in a more continuous manner using an ambulatory system.[23] Improved survival with ambulatory oxygen might result from the increased oxygen duration, that is, they receive oxygen for a greater portion of the day, or it may be a result of the methodology itself. Ambulatory oxygen administration allows many patients to have increased exercise capabilities and to participate in normal activities of daily living, including social pursuits. Thus, it is distinctly possible that the benefits accrued from ambulatory oxygen result from both the *method* and *duration* of therapy delivery. These aspects are considered in more detail in chapter 7.

Pulmonary rehabilitation programme organisation

The staffing and structure of a pulmonary rehabilitation programme can vary tremendously.[26–29] Currently, the great majority of pulmonary rehabilitation programmes are outpatient based for practical and economic reasons. Inpatient programmes are much more expensive and tend to foster the dependency needs of patients. Exceptions to such programmes are patients who need to undergo pulmonary rehabilitation before lung transplantation, which is a subject that goes beyond the scope of this chapter (see chapter 11). Suffice it to say that pulmonary rehabilitation, both before and after lung transplantation, is an important adjunct to this care but only pertains to a small minority of patients who have chronic respiratory disease states.

Every successful pulmonary rehabilitation programme has its "spiritual leader"—often a nurse or respiratory therapist who organises and coordinates all the activities of the programme. A medical director is required in most programmes and sometimes takes the leadership role, but quite often this is not the case.

Staff usually include one or more additional individuals who could be respiratory therapists, nurses, physical therapists, social workers, or indeed anyone with an interest in human beings who is willing to learn the fundamentals of pulmonary rehabilitation.

Most programmes enrol patients in small groups of four to six, and can range in length from four to eight weeks. The initial sessions focus on goals, objectives, anatomy, physiology, and drugs used in pulmonary rehabilitation. Later sessions focus on breathing re-training, breathing exercises, and systemic exercise. Although treadmills and bicycle ergometers are commonly used, they are not necessary and, at times, not very palatable for patients who have limited exercise capabilities. As exercise training is task specific, improving bicycle riding may not be translated into better activities of daily living. Riding a bicycle or walking on a treadmill will allow for the calculation of work accomplished, but the skills required for these kinds of exercise training may not be possessed by every patient. Normal walking in halls, corridors, or outside, often over a measured course, is a more suitable and practical approach to exercise in most patients. What is taught in pulmonary rehabilitation is the method of breathing and exercising, rather than the accomplishment of training itself.

Daily exercise is continued at home to achieve maximum benefit, and it must be continued or the benefit is quickly lost. The great majority of patients can walk longer and sometimes faster at a lower respiratory rate and lower heart rate, with lower oxygen consumption and lower carbon dioxide production. As numerous studies have established that these objectives can be met by most patients, such measurements are not needed in the ordinary course of a pulmonary rehabilitation programme unless research questions are being asked.

Most programmes have social support groups which are critically important to the continued success of the rehabilitation process. Patient newsletters, monthly luncheons with informative lectures, and social outings such as bus or train trips, cruises, and annual celebrations in the form of rallies, have become the hallmark of the most successful programmes in the United States of America.

Outcome of pulmonary rehabilitation

It is virtually impossible to design prospective controlled clinical trials to test the outcome of pulmonary rehabilitation in terms of survival, because any comparative group would require an equal duration of intervention such as music therapy, sun bathing, or other diversionary activities, to act as a control for the additional attention and social interaction provided to patients during a

Table 1.1 Background factors of patients participating in a rehabilitation programme in Denver*

| | Emphysema | | |
	Rehabilitation	Registry	p
No. of men	72	72	—
Age (years)	58·5	58·9	NS
Height (cm)	175	175	—
FEV$_1$ (l/s)	1·08	1·15	NS
Sao_2 (%)†	89	88	NS

* Compared with patients studied in the same laboratory, but treated by their private physicians.
† Breathing air.

pulmonary rehabilitation programme. There would also be a high probability that a self selection process would develop with more motivated individuals choosing the more active intervention that is available.

Comparison of survival curves of patients participating in a pulmonary rehabilitation programme, although interesting, also do not give a firm answer about the impact on survival of such a programme. In the late 1960s and early 1970s, our group matched 72 men who were participating in a pulmonary rehabilitation programme with 72 patients who had equal degrees of emphysema but who were receiving care from their personal physician in Denver (Table 1.1). This was not a randomised prospective clinical trial, but rather a simple comparison of survival of matched groups of patients who lived in the same environment, although some historical controls were included. Patients in the pulmonary rehabilitation study were from a lower socioeconomic group than the control patients. It is generally acknowledged that survival relates to socioeconomic status, and in fact the survival curves are quite similar with a slightly better outcome in the pulmonary rehabilitation group ($p = 0·08$) (Figure 1.1). Although these survival curves have been widely published, they cannot be taken as proof of improved survival as a result of a pulmonary rehabilitation programme.

Some time ago the author's group analysed the outcome of a large number of patients who entered a pulmonary rehabilitation programme at a community hospital, to obtain survival data in the late 1970s and early 1980s. Results of this analysis have been published elsewhere[30] and have been presented at an international

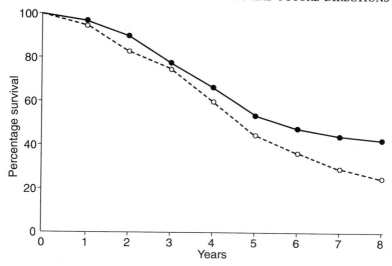

Figure 1.1 Comparison of survival curves of emphysema registered patients versus rehabilitation study patients (all men). (●) Rehabilitated; (−−−) emphysema registered; $n = 72$.

conference on pulmonary rehabilitation.[31] Table 1.2 lists the background factors of 240 patients who were followed for up to nine years, and Figure 1.2 presents the actuarial survival curve from this population. Although these outcome data are not compared with any control groups, they do show a fairly favourable outcome, considering the age and the severity of airflow obstruction observed in the patients who participated in this study. The approximate 40% survival at nine years is similar to that from the data presented in Figure 1.1. Table 1.3 lists the age and sex at time of death. Then it is apparent that these patients died in their late 60s, which indicates fairly good longevity for the selected patients in this study.

Two reviews of the outcome of pulmonary rehabilitation have been published,[32] and citations of additional survivor data are given. A well designed, randomised, controlled, clinical trial compared the results of a comprehensive pulmonary rehabilitation programme which emphasised daily exercise with a control group who received only an education programme together with the usual care.[33] The pulmonary rehabilitation patients achieved a significantly greater maximal exercise tolerance compared with the control group. The

Table 1.2   Background factors of study group $(n=240)$*

No. (%) of men	129 (53·7)
No. (%) of women	111 (46·3)
Average age at entry:	
Total group	64·9 ± 8·03
Men	65·3 ± 8·05
Women	64·5 ± 8·01
FVC	2·02 ± 0·71
FEV_1	
Pre	0·89 ± 0·37
Post	0·97 ± 0·38
Po_2	66·04 ± 11·62
Pco_2	41·8 ± 7·97
Height (cm)	167·58 ± 11·3
Weight (kg)	65·9 ± 15·3
Smoking (packs/year) $(n=221)$	60·77 ± 37·67

Table 3   Age and gender at death

	n	Age (years)		Mean survival (years)
		Range	SD	
Men	69	69·5	±8·10	5·6
Women	36	68·9	±6·75	4·8

follow up was for six years and this revealed a trend towards improved survival and fewer hospitalisations that was not statistically significant.[33] The exercise benefits were partially maintained for at least one year with monthly reinforcements, and tended to diminish after that.[33]

Importance of early identification and intervention

COPD results in an insidious attack upon alveoli and small airways, which covers a timespan of about 30 years, so early identification and intervention appear to be the key to altering its course and prognosis. It is now established that simple measures of airflow abnormality, including a reduction in FEV_1 and FEV_1 as a percentage of the FVC, accurately predict a population of patients who are at risk of premature losses of ventilatory function[34]—accelerated losses of ventilatory function correlate with adverse outcomes in COPD.

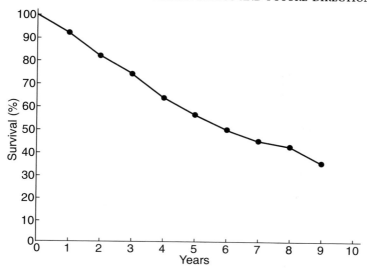

Figure 1.2 Survival of consecutive patients ($n=240$) who entered a pulmonary rehabilitation programme in the 1970s and 1980s. (Reprinted with permission from Burns et al.[30])

The ability to stop smoking has been shown to alter the rate of decline of ventilatory function, particularly in younger individuals with only modest degrees of airflow abnormality.[35] Certainly, such studies can be taken as important indicators of benefit from early identification and intervention through smoking cessation. Currently, as mentioned earlier, there is a great interest in techniques of smoking cessation which include behavioural modification, choice of a quit date, and use of nicotine replacement for the most addicted individuals. Other drugs such as clonidine and certain tranquillisers may relieve nicotine withdrawal symptoms.

The results of a major multicentre trial in the United States of America, known as the Lung Health Study, have been published;[36] the study focused on the impact of early identification and intervention in smokers with mild to moderate forms of COPD. In all, 10 centres enrolled 5887 patients into a prospective study which was designed to compare outcomes of special care, including behavioural modification and smoking cessation, with ordinary care.[36 37] A subset of patients in the special care group also received a bronchodilator, ipratropium bromide, designed to deal with non-specific bronchial hyperreactivity, which has been shown to be an

11

adverse prognostic factor in the decline of ventilatory function in mild to moderate stages of disease. Thirty seven per cent of those enrolled in this study were women. It has already been shown that women have a greater degree of bronchial hyperreactivity than men with otherwise equal background factors,[37] so whether or not this can be reduced with the long term use of ipratropium and anticholinergic bronchodilator remains to be seen.

The Lung Health Study showed striking differences in the rate of decline in FEV_1 in those patients who were randomised to receive special care. Special care offered a more intensive programme aimed at smoking cessation. Almost 40% of the special care patients ceased to smoke at some time during the five year follow up compared with the usual care patients who only achieved a quit rate of about 20% at any time during the follow up. Sustained quitters were 22% from the special care group versus 5% from the usual care group. The rate of decline in FEV_1 was far slower in the special care group, suggesting a favourable effect on prognosis. Although a measurable response to inhaled ipratropium was maintained during the follow up, there were no changes in the baseline FEV_1 in the ipratropium group, indicating no basic improvement in course and prognosis in response to ipratropium, although this does not negate any beneficial symptomatic benefit.

Although cause of death was not a primary outcome objective, Table 1.4 shows some interesting results: 57 of the study patients died from lung cancer compared with only 37 from cardiovascular causes (heart attack and stroke deaths). This is a striking observation considering the relatively young age of the participants (mean age 48·5 years). No patient died of COPD during the follow

Table 4 Causes of death: five year follow up of 5877 patients in Lung Health Study*

	Special intervention plus ipratropium	Special intervention plus placebo	Usual care	Total
Lung cancer	18	20	19	57
Coronary heart disease/ cardiovascular disease	18	7	12	37
Other	18	17	20	55
Total	54	44	51	149

* Mean age 48·5 ± 6·8 years.
Modified from Anthonisen et al.[36]

up because of the mild nature of the disease of those involved. This study now underscores the profound value of measuring spirometry in patients with only mild airflow obstruction because it identifies a population at high risk of developing lung cancer.[38-41]

Finally, some musings based entirely on clinical observations about the basic nature of COPD. Consider the hypothesis that COPD should be considered as a constitutionally determined multiorgan system disease state.[42] Whether or not this hypothesis explains the multiplicity of factors that conspire to create the pathophysiological state of COPD—a process that takes 30–40 years and culminates with premature morbidity and mortality—remains to be established.[42]

It may be appropriate to consider COPD as a multisystem disease for the following reasons. Patients who have any stage of COPD exhibit a common affective disorder which is characterised by anxiety, depression, and somatic preoccupation. Anxiety and depression can be reduced with tobacco use, which may be one of the main reasons why nicotine addiction in COPD patients is so strong. In addition, smokers on average weigh less than non-smokers; they tend to consume foods higher in fat and cholesterol and lower in fibre and antioxidant vitamins. Deficiency in antioxidant vitamins may be an additional factor in the premature morbidity and mortality that occur in COPD patients.[42] Also there is an intriguing lack of physical fitness in men compared with women with only mild abnormalities in airflow.[43 44] Accordingly it may be wise to consider dietary changes and the use of antioxidant vitamins and physical conditioning early in the course of COPD, at least in men.

Conclusion

Pulmonary rehabilitation is an established method of care for patients with advanced COPD and related pulmonary disorders. Pulmonary rehabilitation goes beyond ordinary care and involves patient and family education, breathing training, systemic exercises, and patient support groups. All patients enrolled in a pulmonary rehabilitation programme require the systematic use of both bronchoactive and strategic drugs. Oxygen is life saving in selected patients with chronic stable hypoxaemia. Pulmonary rehabilitation improves the quality of life and probably extends useful life, and should be considered the standard of care for patients who wish to receive more than ordinary care.

1 Petty TL. Pulmonary rehabilitation. *Am Rev Respir Dis* 1980;**122**:159–61.
2 Petty TL, Nett LM. *Enjoying life with emphysema*, 3rd edn. Cedar Grove, New York: Laemmec Publishing, 1995: 199.
3 Ramsdell JW, Nachtwey FJ, Moser KM. Bronchial hyperreactivity in chronic obstructive bronchitis. *Am Rev Respir Dis* 1982;**126**:829–32.
4 Braun SR, McKenzie WN, Copeland C, *et al*. A comparison of the effect of ipratropium and albuterol in the treatment of chronic obstructive airway disease. *Arch Intern Med* 1989;**149**:544–7.
5 Murciano D, Auclair MH, Pariento R, *et al*. A randomized, controlled trial of theophylline in patients with severe chronic obstructive pulmonary disease. *N Engl J Med* 1989;**320**:1521–5.
6 Albert RK, Martin TR, Lewis RW. Controlled clinical trial of methylprednisolone in patients with chronic bronchitis and acute respiratory insufficiency. *Ann Intern Med* 1980;**92**:753–8.
7 Postma DS, Steenhuis EJ, van der Weele LT, *et al*. Severe chronic airflow obstruction: can corticosteroids slow down progression? *Eur J Respir Dis* 1985;**67**:56–64.
8 Postma DS, Peters I, Steenhuis EJ, *et al*. Moderately severe chronic airflow obstruction. Can corticosteroids slow down obstruction? *Eur Respir J* 1988;**1**:22–6.
9 Mendella LA, Manfreda J, Warren CP, *et al*. Steroid response in stable chronic obstructive pulmonary disease. *Ann Intern Med* 1982;**96**:17–21.
10 Pride NB, Vermeire P, Allegra L. Diagnostic labels applied to model case histories of chronic airflow obstruction. Responses to a questionnaire in 11 North American and Western European Countries. *Eur Respir J* 1989;**2**:702–9.
11 Petty TL. The National Mucolytic Study. Results of a randomized, double-blind, placebo-controlled study of iodinated glycerol in chronic obstructive bronchitis. *Chest* 1990;**97**:75–83.
12 Anthonisen NR, Manfreda J, Warren CP, *et al*. Antibiotic therapy in exacerbations of chronic obstructive pulmonary disease. *Ann Intern Med* 1987;**106**:196–204.
13 Transdermal Nicotine Study Group. Transdermal nicotine for smoking cessation. Six-month results from two multicenter controlled clinical trials. *JAMA* 1991;**266**:3133–8.
14 Recommendations of ACIP. Prevention and control of influenza. *Morbidity and Mortality Weekly Report* 1984;**34**:261–75.
15 Immunization Practices Advisory Committee. Update: pneumococcal polysaccharide vaccine usage—United States. *Morbidity and Mortality Weekly Report* 1984;**33**:273–6.
16 Mueller RE, Petty TL, Filley GF. Ventilation and arterial blood gas changes induced by pursed lips breathing. *J Appl Physiol* 1970;**28**:784–9.
17 Tiep BL, Burns MR, Kao O, *et al*. Pursed lips breathing training using ear oximeter. *Chest* 1986;**90**:218–21.
18 Anderson JB, Dragsted L, Kann T, *et al*. Resistive breathing training in severe chronic obstructive pulmonary disease—a pilot study. *Scand J Respir Dis* 1979;**60**:151–6.
19 Pardy RL, Rivington RN, Despas PJ, *et al*. The effects of inspiratory muscle training on exercise performance in chronic airflow limitation. *Am Rev Respir Dis* 1981;**123**:426–33.

20 Belman MJ. Exercise in chronic obstructive pulmonary disease. *Clin Chest Med* 1986;7:585–97.

21 Guthrie AG, Petty TL. Improved exercise tolerance in patients with chronic airway obstruction. *Phys Ther* 1970;50:1333–7.

22 Casaburi R, Patessio A, Ioli F, *et al.* Reductions in exercise lactic acidosis and ventilation as a result of exercise training in patients with obstructive lung disease. *Am Rev Respir Dis* 1991;143:9–18.

23 Nocturnal Oxygen Therapy Trial Group. Continuous or nocturnal oxygen therapy in hypoxemic chronic obstructive lung disease: A clinical trial. *Ann Intern Med* 1980;93:391–8.

24 Report of the Medical Research Council Working Party. Long term domiciliary oxygen therapy in chronic cor pulmonale complicating chronic bronchitis and emphysema. *Lancet* 1981;i:681–6.

25 Casaburi R, Petty TL (eds). *Principles and practice of pulmonary rehabilitation.* Philadelphia: WB Saunders, 1993:508.

26 Tiep BL. Pulmonary rehabilitation program organization. In Casaburi R, Petty TL (eds), *Principles and practice of pulmonary rehabilitation.* Philadelphia: WB Saunders, 1993:302–16.

27 Tietsort J. A storefront program for pulmonary rehabilitation. In Casaburi R, Petty TL (eds), *Principles and practice of pulmonary rehabilitation.* Philadelphia: WB Saunders, 1993:474–7.

28 Sutton FD. The proprietary pulmonary rehabilitation program. In Casaburi R, Petty (eds), *Principles and practice of pulmonary rehabilitation.* Philadelphia: WB Saunders, 1993:478–82.

29 Kravetz HM. How the office-based pulmonary rehabilitation works. In Casaburi R, Petty TL (eds), *Principles and practice of pulmonary rehabilitation.* Philadelphia: WB Saunders, 1993:483–6.

30 Burns MR, Sherman B, Madison R, *et al.* Pulmonary rehabilitation outcome. *Respiratory Therapy* 1989;2:25–30.

31 Petty TL. Pulmonary rehabilitation: Historical roots, present status, and future directions. Presented at the Annual Meeting of the Hong Kong Thoracic Society, 22 April 1993.

32 Clark CJ. Evaluating the results of pulmonary rehabilitation treatment. In Casaburi R, Petty TL (eds), *Principles and practice of pulmonary rehabilitation.* Philadelphia: WB Saunders, 1993.

33 Ries AL, Kaplan RM, Linberg TM, *et al.* Effects of pulmonary rehabilitation and physiologic and psychological outcomes in patients with COPD. *Ann Intern Med* 1995;122:823–32.

34 Burrows B, Knudson RJ, Camilli AE, *et al.* The "horse racing effect" and predicting decline in forced expiratory volume in one-second from screening spirometry. *Am Rev Respir Dis* 1987;135:788–93.

35 Peto R, Speizer FE, Cochrane AL, *et al.* The relevance in adults of airflow obstruction, but not of mucus hypersecretion, to mortality from chronic lung disease. *Am Rev Resir Dis* 1983;128:491–500.

36 Anthonisen NR, Connett JE, Kiley JP, *et al.* Effects of smoking intervention and the use of an inhaled anticholinergic bronchodilator on the rate of decline of FEV_1. The Lung Health Study. *JAMA* 1994;272:1497–505.

37 Tashkin DP, Altose MD, Bleecker ER, *et al.* The lung health study: Airway responsiveness to inhaled methacholine in smokers with mild to moderate airflow limitation. The Lung Health Study Research Group. *Am Rev Respir Dis* 1992;145:301–10.

38 Skillrud DM, Offord KP, Miller RD. Higher risk of lung cancer in chronic obstructive pulmonary disease. *Ann Intern Med* 1986;105:503–7.

39 Tockman MS, Anthonisen NR, Wright EC, *et al.* Airways obstruction and the risk for lung cancer. *Ann Intern Med* 1987;106:512–18.

40 Kuller LH, Ockene J, Meilahn E, *et al.* Relation of forced expiratory volume in one second (FEV$_1$) to lung cancer mortality in the Multiple Risk Factor Intervention Trial (MRFIT). *Am J Epidemiol* 1990;**132**:265–74.
41 Nomura A, Stemmerman GN, Chyou P, *et al.* Prospective study of pulmonary function and lung cancer. *Am Rev Respir Dis* 1991;**144**:307–11.
42 Petty TL. Pulmonary rehabilitation of early COPD: COPD as a systemic disease (editorial). *Chest* 1994;**105**:1636–7.
43 Carter R, Nicrota B, Blevins W, *et al.* Altered exercise gas exchange and cardiac function in patients with mild chronic obstructive pulmonary disease. *Chest* 1993;**1034**:745–50.
44 Carter R, Nicrota B, Huber G. Differing effects of airway obstruction on physical work capacity and ventilation in men and women with COPD. *Chest* 1994;**106**:1730–9.

2 Exercise in patients with COPD

MICHAEL J BELMAN

Exercise is widely promoted as a means of improving physical endurance. It is recommended, not only for the healthy, but also for individuals with various disabilities and disease. In respiratory medicine we have witnessed several decades of investigation directed not only at the pathophysiology of exercise in patients with chronic obstructive pulmonary disease (COPD), but also at the effects of exercise training in improving function. As was initially the case with coronary artery disease, many physicians of the mid-twentieth century adopted a very conservative approach and generally discouraged exercise in patients with significant COPD. Despite the pleas for greater physical exercise for patients with chronic lung disease by Barach, a pioneer of pulmonary medicine,[1] it was only in the late 1960s and early 1970s that his ideas were aggressively pursued. In the United States of America there is now widespread support for pulmonary rehabilitation programmes which, almost without exception, include a liberal dose of exercise training. The transfer of the standard recommendations for exercise training to healthy subjects and even cardiac patients has not been easy. The pattern of exercise response in patients with COPD presents some unusual and, in some cases, unique features that require radical rethinking of the traditional advice given to the normal subject and those with heart disease. The purpose of this review is to highlight key features of the pathophysiology of this exercise pattern in patients with COPD and to analyse the evidence which supports exercise training.

Exercise limitation in COPD

Abnormalities of ventilatory mechanics, respiratory muscles, alveolar gas exchange, and cardiac function are present to varying degrees in patients with COPD. Delineation of the major mechanisms underlying exercise limitation has obvious value in that treatment aimed at reducing the severity of a major limiting factor would be beneficial in improving exercise function. This process has not always been easy and it is likely that the importance of limiting factors is not the same in every patient. The discussion below deals with each of these factors separately, although they are probably interrelated in most patients.

Ventilation and pulmonary mechanics

This is one of the most important factors that limits exercise performance. Expiratory air flow obstruction is the main pathophysiological result of the alveolar wall destruction and bronchiolar narrowing which characterises this disease. In moderate to severe obstructive lung disease resting expiratory airflows approach or are equal to maximal airflow.[2 3] In contrast to normal subjects in whom expiratory flow limitation may only occur during expiration at the highest work rates, patients with COPD show flow limitation over most or all of expiration at low exercise levels (Figure 2.1). In patients with severe disease flow limitation is present at rest.[4] The prolongation of expiration together with a higher than normal exercise breathing frequency leads inexorably to dynamic hyperinflation with an increase in end expiratory lung volume.[5] The dynamic hyperinflation causes an increase in inspiratory loading and work through:

1 A decrease in static compliance as patients now breathe along a shallower portion of the pressure–volume curve
2 A high inspiratory threshold load caused by the need to generate additional pressure required to overcome elastic recoil pressure before inspiratory flow can begin (this increased threshold pressure has been referred to as intrinsic positive end expiratory pressure)
3 An exaggeration of dependence of compliance on frequency.

As Younes[5] has stated: "While the mechanical defect is primarily resistive in nature in expiration, the mechanical consequences are encountered in inspiration and are primarily restrictive in nature."

18

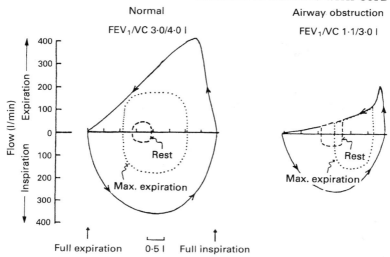

Figure 2.1   Spontaneous flow–volume curves at rest (dotted lines) and maximum exercise (dashed lines) as well as maximum flow–volume curves at rest (outer solid line) in a normal subject and a patient with chronic airway obstruction. (Reproduced with permission from Gallagher.[2])

The more severe the reduction in the forced expiratory volume in one second (FEV_1), the greater the increase in end expiratory lung volume.[6] The dynamic hyperinflation brings with it an increase in inspiratory load, but it is a necessary evil for without it the patients with COPD would not be able to increase ventilation to meet the demands of exercise. As end expiratory lung volume rises the patient is able to increase maximum expiratory airflow by breathing along a higher portion of the expiratory flow–volume curve.[47]

The importance of end expiratory lung volume in patients with mild COPD (FEV_1/FVC ratios of about 60%) has recently been emphasised.[8] In these patients it was thought that ventilatory limitation plays only a minor part in contrast to patients with more severe disease. In a recent study, however, it was shown that, although the ratio of maximum exercise ventilation ($\dot{V}E$max) to the maximum voluntary ventilation at peak exercise was considerably less than 70%—a value traditionally used to rule out a ventilatory limitation—these patients demonstrated a rise in end expiratory lung volume and flow limitation during exercise. In contrast, age matched control subjects maintained or reduced their resting end expiratory lung volume and achieved a maximum oxygen consumption ($\dot{V}o_2$max) which was 30% higher than that of the patients. These investigators concluded that, despite the mild degree of COPD, there was a significant impact on pulmonary mechanics during exercise.[8]

Because the respiratory system in the exercising patient with COPD fails to reach its relaxation volume, inspiration can only occur after respiratory muscles develop sufficient force to overcome the recoil pressure of the hyperinflated chest. Preliminary studies have now examined the effect of apply continuous positive airway pressure as a means of providing inspiratory assistance.[9 10] The results of this work showed that continuous positive airway pressure reduced the work of breathing and dyspnoea. In the study by O'Donnell and colleagues[9] the exercise endurance was prolonged. This response emphasises the importance of negating the loading effect of the intrinsic positive end expiratory pressure.

Dodd and colleagues[11] have shown that patients with airflow obstruction attempt to compensate for the increase in end expiratory lung volume by actively recruiting abdominal and expiratory rib cage muscles during expiration. At the onset of inspiration the patients rapidly relaxed these muscles, an effect that allows them to exploit the outward recoil of the chest wall and gravitational descent of the diaphragm at the onset of inspiration. This reaction functions as a form of inspiratory assistance. On the other hand, excessive use of expiratory musculature during expiration increases oxygen utilisation of the expiratory muscles, further reducing the overall efficiency of breathing in these patients.[12]

It is well recognised that in moderate to severe COPD maximal exercise ventilation reaches a high percentage of the maximum ventilatory ventilation (MVV) at rest. This $\dot{V}$Emax/MVV ratio may in fact even exceed 100% in patients with severe airflow obstruction.[13] There are significant correlations between measures of expiratory airflow such as the FEV_1 and MVV on the one hand, and $\dot{V}$Emax and $\dot{V}o_2$max on the other.[14 15] Because of the relatively large scatter of the data, however, the confidence intervals of individual predictions are large and it is not possible to predict peak minute ventilation with great accuracy in an individual patient. For example, the 95% confidence interval of one equation is ± 18 l/min despite a correlation coefficient of 0·97.[14] Factors other than mechanical ventilatory limitation also have a role (see below).

20

Respiratory muscle dysfunction

Patients with COPD exhibit respiratory muscle weakness (see Tobin[16] for review). Intrinsic factors such as hypoxia, hypercapnia, acidaemia, and malnutrition impair respiratory muscle contactility. Superimposed on this are the mechanical derangements which further weaken diaphragmatic function. Hyperinflation shortens the diaphragm, moving it to a disadvantageous portion of its length–tension curve. Moreover, the zone of apposition is reduced and this impairs the optimal inspiratory action of the muscle (Figure 2.2).[16] Although patients with COPD show compensatory changes in the diaphragm which allow for relative preservation of function even at the limits of hyperinflation,[17] these inspiratory pressures are still well below those of normal subjects at functional residual capacity (FRC).[18] Activity of the upper limbs[19 20] is an additional aggravating factor which hampers diaphragmatic function. During arm work the stabilising effect of the shoulder girdle on the thorax is lost and the inspiratory load is shifted onto the diaphragm and muscles of expiration. In these circumstances the diaphragm is required to assume a greater load and, as noted above, is ill prepared to do so (Figure 2.3).[19 20] The net result is a greater limitation of arm than of leg exercise associated with the earlier onset of dyspnoea in many patients with severe airflow obstruction. As performance of most activities of daily living require repetitive

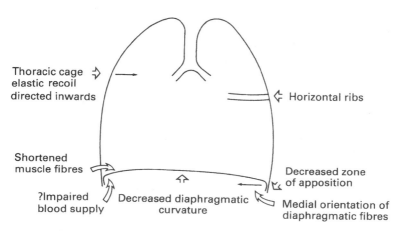

Thoracic cage elastic recoil directed inwards

Horizontal ribs

Shortened muscle fibres

Decreased zone of apposition

?Impaired blood supply

Decreased diaphragmatic curvature

Medial orientation of diaphragmatic fibres

Figure 2.2   Detrimental effect of hyperinflation on respiratory muscle function. (Reproduced with permission from Tobin.[16])

21

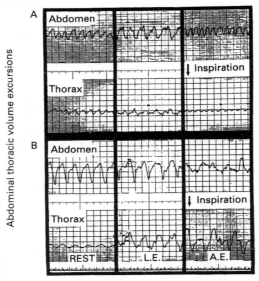

Time (seconds)

Figure 2.3   Tracings of abdominal and thoracic excursions. Panel A shows excursions in a patient with synchronous thoracoabdominal movements at rest during leg exercise (LE) and arm exercise (AE). Panel B shows that the synchronous pattern observed at rest and during LE changes to dyssynchronous during AE. Full inward retraction during inspection is seen in the last two breaths of the arm exercise tracing. (Reproduced with permission from Celli et al.[19])

upper extremity movement, this phenomenon has important implications for patients with COPD (see Upper limb exercise training below).

Respiratory muscle fatigue

Whether or not respiratory muscle fatigue occurs during exercise in patients with COPD is not clear. Preliminary evidence from Pardy and coworkers[21] showed that in some patients a decrease in the high to low ratio—an electromyographic index of fatigue—occurred in only some patients during exercise. The fact that the high to low ratio has proved useful in carefully controlled laboratory experiments does not imply that it can be transferred to use in individuals during exercise. As Younes has stated,[22] a change in the ratio may occur between rest and exercise because of changes in breathing pattern and changes in the spatial relationship of the electromyographic electrode and the muscle. Moreover, other muscles recruited at higher exercise intensities may contaminate the signal. The presence of thoracoabdominal asynchrony during breathing has also been cited as support for the presence of inspiratory muscle fatigue. More recent evidence[23][24] indicates, however, that asynchrony of the thorax and abdomen during inspiration is not pathognomonic of fatigue, but may be seen in circumstances in which an individual breathes against a high inspiratory load. With cessation of the loading the breathing pattern returns to normal, even though presumably the low frequency fatigue induced by the loading persists for several additional hours. Definitive proof of fatigue would require documentation of decreased muscle contractility after performance of work. Rochester has emphasised that inspiratory muscle weakness is more important than fatigue.[18][25] He emphasises the ratio of the pressure required per breath to the maximum inspiratory pressure (Pbreath/Pmax) as an index of the weakness. During exercise Pbreath rises as inspiratory work increases while the rise in end expiratory lung volume and configurational changes in the diaphragm reduce the Pmax. The net effect is a reduction in functional diaphragmatic strength during exercise.

Impaired gas exchange

Hypoxaemia, a common feature of COPD, frequently shows further reductions during exercise. A low diffusing capacity (<55% of the predicted value) has been used as a predictor of those patients in whom exercise desaturation will occur.[26] The hypoxaemia of exercise is largely due to the effects of a reduction in mixed venous Po$_2$ on low ventilation diffusion lung units[27] aggravated in some cases by hypoventilation. On the other hand, some patients do show an improvement in Pao$_2$ with exercise which must reflect an improvement in intrapulmonary ventilation–perfusion matching.[28] There is little evidence for diffusion limitation. The absence of the normal exercise decrease in the physiological dead space to tidal volume ratio (Vd/Vt) further aggravates the ventilatory limitation in COPD. In order to maintain efficient carbon dioxide output in the presence of a reduced alveolar ventilation, greater than normal increases in total minute ventilation are required as exercise intensity increases[29] (see Lactic acidosis and exercise training below).

Cardiovascular function

Remodelling of the muscular arteries and arterioles is the main cause of the increase in pulmonary vascular resistance.[30] These changes lead to thickening of the intima and narrowing of the arterial and arteriolar lumina and are more extensive than the increase in muscle seen in the media of medium and small arteries in people exposed to high altitude hypoxia. Other factors that play a part in the elevated pulmonary vascular pressures include emphysematous destruction of the vascular bed, alveolar hypoxia, increased alveolar pressure, increased haematocrit, and acidosis.[31]

Commonly observed abnormalities of cardiovascular function during exercise are an increased heart rate/$\dot{V}o_2$ ratio related to a shift upwards and to the left of the heart rate/$\dot{V}o_2$ slope which itself, however, may be normal.[2 32] In other words, at a comparable $\dot{V}o_2$ the heart rate in a patient with COPD is increased with a corresponding decrease in the oxygen pulse. This means that estimation of exercise intensity in these patients by means of heart rate can be erroneous (Figure 2.4).[33] A heart rate of 120–130 beats/

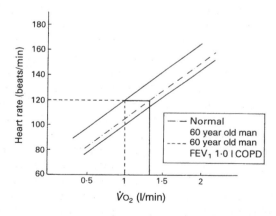

Figure 2.4   Normal heart rate response to exercise is illustrated by the parallel solid lines. In the patient with COPD, in whom the heart response is generally at the upper limit of normal, the $\dot{V}o_2$ achieved at a heart rate of 120 beats/min (1·0 l/min) would be less than a normal subject (1·33 l/min).

min in a normal individual reflects a $\dot{V}o_2$ of greater than 1 litre/min whereas in a patient with COPD this may represent a significantly lower $\dot{V}o_2$. This phenomenon has implications for the intensity of exercise training which will be discussed later. The reduction in heart rates achieved at peak exercise are proportionately less than the reduction in peak $\dot{V}o_2$, and the maximal oxygen pulse at peak exercise is therefore smaller. The rise in the cardiac output/$\dot{V}o_2$ relationship is considered generally to be normal[2] despite the fact that pulmonary vascular resistance is increased and there is a higher than normal rise in pulmonary artery pressure. The increased afterload on the right ventricle can cause right ventricular dysfunction, but whether or not this actually limits exercise is unclear.[31]

Lactic acidosis

Lactic acid is produced during incremental exercise although the time at which it appears in arterial blood varies and is dependent on circulatory function and level of fitness. The point at which blood lactate rises has been termed the lactic acid threshold and precedes, by about 150 ml of $\dot{V}o_2$, the increase in minute ventilation related to the increased carbon dioxide output.[34 35] This increase in ventilation can be detected by one of many indices as described by Wasserman and coworkers but, most recently, they have emphasised the use of the "V slope criterion".[36] In this index the rate of rise in carbon dioxide output is plotted against oxygen uptake. Although oxygen uptake remains linear at the onset of lactic acid production, carbon dioxide output increases and so a break point can be discerned. This inflection point has been termed the "anaerobic threshold" by Wasserman and colleagues, whereas other investigators have used the term "ventilation threshold". This difference in terminology symbolises a heated controversy. Wasserman et al feel that the appearance of lactic acid truly indicates a transition to anaerobic glycolysis because of tissue hypoxia.[37] Their critics disagree and consider that, although lactic acid certainly does rise during exercise, it does not necessarily imply anaerobiosis but merely an imbalance between lactate production on the one hand and its utilisation on the other.[38] In patients with COPD lactic acid and anaerobic thresholds can be determined even in those with moderately severe disease[39] although, clearly, peak lactate levels will be considerably reduced in these patients because of their overall reduction in exercise capacity.[39 40] It should be noted

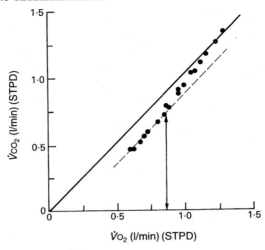

Figure 2.5 Carbon dioxide output ($\dot{V}CO_2$) plotted against oxygen uptake ($\dot{V}O_2$). When the anaerobic threshold is reached, $\dot{V}CO_2$ accelerates compared with $\dot{V}O_2$. The inflection point marking this acceleration is shown by the arrow. (Reproduced with permission from Sue *et al.*[39])

that the lactic acid in these patients probably arises from working limb muscles because it is those patients who reach the highest work rates who show the highest lactate levels.[40] Conversely, patients with very severe obstructive disease in whom respiratory muscle work is high have low lactate levels and, moreover, lactate levels during isocapnic hyperpnoea are only marginally increased.[41]

Sue *et al*[39] feel that the V slope criterion is useful in detecting metabolic acidosis in these patients (Figure 2.5) but recognition of V slope may not always be easy, as was shown in a study[42] in which not only was there considerable interobserver variability in V slope detection but a significant number of patients with exercise induced metabolic acidosis did not develop inflection points. Conversely, inflection points were found in patients without metabolic acidosis. This finding detracts from the value of the V slope in detecting metabolic acidosis in patients with COPD (see Exercise training below).

Peripheral muscle fatigue

Despite the emphasis on impaired ventilatory mechanics and dyspnoea it is now well documented that a significant number of

26

patients with COPD will stop exercising because of peripheral muscle fatigue.[43] In a recent study about one third of patients stopped for this reason. In addition, both limb and respiratory muscle show parallel decrements in strength and contribute independently to reduced exercise capacity.

These are the major pathophysiological abnormalities seen in COPD, but other factors do play a part in limiting exercise. Their recognition is important as treatment aimed at improving functional capacity must take them into account. Additional factors include nutritional status through its effect on both limb and respiratory muscle strength and endurance,[44] perception of and response to breathlessness which varies among patients,[45 46] and psychological factors such as depression, anxiety, and fear of exercise.[47] Furthermore, the role of deconditioning—a common problem in these patients because of their chronic inactivity—can aggravate the impaired exercise tolerance.[40] Although breathlessness is clearly related to the severity of abnormalities in expiratory air flow this is not the only factor, as recently emphasised by O'Donnell *et al*[48] who showed that patients with comparable levels of airway obstruction may have varying degrees of breathlessness. The major differences between mildly and severely breathless patients were the presence of hypoxaemia during exercise and an abnormally low diffusing capacity in the second group. Other investigators have shown an additional effect of psychological and psychosocial factors on functional capacity over and above that of lung function. Their analyses showed that dyspnoea, respiratory muscle strength, and spirometry each contributed independently to functional limitation and emphasised that each of them should be assessed separately.[45]

Exercise training in COPD

Pulmonary rehabilitation programmes vary in their complexity and may include several therapeutic components[49 50] including:

1 Patient and family education
2 Treatment of bronchospasm by means of bronchodilators or reduction in bronchial secretions
3 Treatment of bronchial infections
4 Treatment of congestive heart failure
5 Oxygen therapy

6 Chest physical therapy including breathing technique training
7 Exercise reconditioning
8 Psychosocial therapy and vocational rehabilitation.

Controlled exercise studies

Although exercise reconditioning has long been considered an essential component of the rehabilitation process it is only very recently that a randomised study has confirmed this belief.[51] In this eight week study 119 patients with COPD were randomised either to a comprehensive rehabilitation programme including exercise reconditioning or, alternatively, to an education control programme. The investigators provided education, physical and respiratory therapy, psychosocial support, and supervised exercise training to the treated group whereas the control group received twice weekly classroom instruction in respiratory therapy, lung disease, pharmacology, and diet but did not exercise. Before and after the treatment and after an additional six months, both groups underwent extensive physiological and psychosocial tests. The major finding of this study was that at eight weeks the improvement in exercise endurance as measured by treadmill walking showed a mean increase in treadmill time from 12·5 minutes to 23 minutes compared with an insignificant change from 12 to 13 minutes in the control group. At six months the treated group still maintained a comparable advantage with a treadmill endurance of about 21 minutes compared with 12 minutes in the control group. No difference in the quality of well being scale—a measure of health related quality of life—was noted. This well designed, randomised, controlled study definitively established exercise therapy as an essential component of the pulmonary rehabilitation process.

Relatively few other studies have compared treated and control groups. In the study by Cockcroft and colleagues[52] a treated group of 19 patients was compared with a control group of 20 patients. During training the patients used cycle exercise, rowing machines, and swimming and, in addition, free range walking was performed. This treatment was carried out for six weeks in a rehabilitation centre; patients were subsequently discharged and encouraged to continue walking and stair climbing. The control group was given no special instructions to exercise. The findings showed an increase in 12 minute walking distance and peak exercise $\dot{V}o_2$ and $\dot{V}\text{E}$ in the treated group at two months and these differences were significantly greater than those in the control group. The treated group also showed improvement in general well being and dyspnoea. In a study by McGavin and coworkers[53] training was carried out by stair climbing at home, but the patients were tested with a 12 minute walk. In this study of 24 patients (12 in the exercise group and 12 in a control group) a significant, albeit small, improvement in the 12 minute walking distance was noted. Other notable findings were an increase in stride length in the exercise group but no change in peak $\dot{V}O_2$, heart rate, or minute ventilation as measured during an incremental cycle ergometer test. Additional studies comparing treated and control groups are summarised elsewhere.[49]

Uncontrolled exercise studies

Numerous uncontrolled studies of exercise training have been performed during the past three decades, the results of which have been summarised.[3 33 49 50 54] In this review several more recent studies will be dealt with in detail. Apart from the study of Casaburi and coworkers[40] the findings are similar to those in previous work. These studies do, however, effectively highlight the methods of testing and training, and discuss unresolved issues, including mode and intensity of exercise training.

Lactic acidosis and exercise training

In an editorial published in 1986 Casaburi and Wasserman[55] emphasised the role of carbon dioxide output as the major drive to ventilation during exercise. Recognising the well known relationships between $\dot{V}E$ on the one hand and $\dot{V}CO_2$, arterial PCO_2, and VD/VT ratio on the other, they suggested that aerobic training in patients with COPD would reduce carbon dioxide output and the ventilatory stimulus. The interrelationship of these variables is expressed in the equation:

$$\dot{V}E = \frac{k \times \dot{V}CO_2}{PaCO_2 \ (1 - VD/VT)}$$

where $\dot{V}E$ is expired minute ventilation, $\dot{V}CO_2$ is carbon dioxide output, $PaCO_2$ is partial pressure of arterial carbon dioxide, VD/VT is the physiological dead space to tidal volume ratio, and k is a constant.

29

The lactic acid produced during exercise is buffered mainly by bicarbonate with the generation of carbonic acid which dissociates into carbon dioxide and water. The carbon dioxide produced by the buffering of lactic acid must be excreted by the lungs in addition to carbon dioxide produced by muscle metabolism during exercise. Exercise training delays the rise in blood lactate levels so any delay in lactic acid production will, by reducing the carbon dioxide load, decrease the ventilatory requirements during exercise. The effect of aerobic training and reduction in $\dot{V}E$ during exercise has been well documented in normal subjects by these investigators. At high levels of work near peak $\dot{V}O_2$, large reductions of 30–40 l/min in $\dot{V}E$ can be achieved in normal individuals.[40]

With this rationale in mind, Casaburi and Wasserman from the United States of America, in conjunction with a group of Italian investigators,[40] performed a study in which high and low intensity training was performed in patients with COPD and the effects on lactate production were examined in detail. Exercise testing was performed on a cycle ergometer with breath by breath measurements of gas exchange before and after the training. Arterial blood gas measurements and arterial lactate measurements were also made. The anaerobic threshold was determined by means of the modified V slope technique.[36] Training was performed on a calibrated cycle ergometer five days a week for eight weeks. The high intensity group performed exercise at 45 min/day at an intensity 60% of the difference between the anaerobic threshold and the $\dot{V}O_2$max. The low intensity group exercised at 90% of this level, but the duration was increased so that total work performed in the two groups was similar.

The major results of Casaburi's study were a reduction in the peak $\dot{V}CO_2$ and the maximal ventilatory equivalent for oxygen ($\dot{V}E/\dot{V}O_2$) in the high intensity group. In a test with a high work rate and constant load, the high intensity trained group showed significant reductions in blood lactate, $\dot{V}E$, $\dot{V}CO_2$, $\dot{V}O_2$, and the $\dot{V}E/\dot{V}O_2$ ratio. Heart rate at comparable work rates was reduced. All these findings confirm the development of a true aerobic training effect (Figure 2.6). On the other hand, the group who trained at the low intensity, even though the total work performed was similar, showed smaller changes in these variables. In this group, although the lactate decrease was significant (10%), the decreases in $\dot{V}E$, $\dot{V}CO_2$, and $\dot{V}O_2$ were not significantly different. Furthermore, a significant increase in endurance of exercise at the higher work

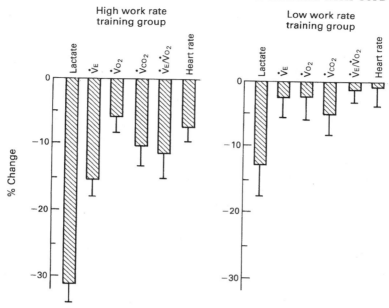

Figure 2.6   Changes in physiological responses to identical exercise tasks in high and low work rate training groups. (Reproduced with permission from Casaburi et al.[40]).

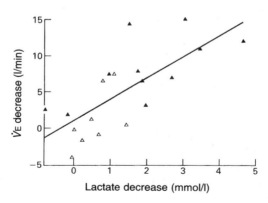

Figure 2.7   Relation between the decrease in ventilation and the decrease in arterial lactate in response to a high constant work rate test as a result of a programme of exercise training: ▲, high work rate trained group; △, low work rate trained group. Solid line is obtained by linear regression. $\Delta \dot{V}_{E_2} = 2 \cdot 84$, Δ [Lactate] $= 1 \cdot 19$. (Reproduced with permission from Casaburi et al.[40])

rate seen in the high intensity trained group (6·6–11·4 min) was not seen in the low intensity trained group (6·9–7·5 min).

There was a significant relationship between the decrease in minute ventilation during exercise and the decrease in blood lactate ($r = 0·73$, $\Delta \dot{V}_E = 2·46$ l/min per mmol lactate). The slope of the relationship $\Delta \dot{V}_E / \Delta$[Lactate] in these patients (Figure 2.7) was considerably lower than that recorded in a previous study in normal subjects in whom the $\dot{V}_E$ decreased by 7·2 l/min per mmol lactate. This study clearly shows that:

1 Significant lactic acidaemia occurs in patients with mild to moderate chronic airway obstruction, and in some cases this may develop at low work rates (pedalling at 0 W)
2 Both high and low intensity training reduce the rise in lactate but the effect with high intensity training is considerably greater
3 Although lactate levels and $\dot{V}_E$ are lower after training in patients with COPD, the reduction in ventilation in patients is only about a third as large as that seen in normal subjects.

The explanation for this difference is related to the fact that these patients show a reduced ventilatory response to the lactic acidosis of exercise and therefore a decrease in lactic acid after training produces a comparably smaller decrease in $\dot{V}_E$.

Although this study clearly shows the generation of a true aerobic training response, this was accomplished in a group of relatively young patients (mean age 49) with rather mild disease (FEV_1 percentage predicted 56% and FEV_1/FVC ratio 58%). These are not the type of patients commonly found in most rehabilitation programmes. In the past most studies examined patients in whom the FEV_1 was considerably lower. In the United States of America it is not unusual to find patients participating in exercise programmes with FEV_1 values of less than 1·01.[49] Moreover, before the training these patients were relatively unfit as shown by the lactate threshold which was found to be at oxygen consumptions below 1 l/min. It is not surprising, therefore, that they responded dramatically to the exercise programmes. The fact that the ventilatory response to exercise acidosis is blunted in patients with COPD further detracts from the practical benefit of lactate reduction. Casaburi et al[40] document a $\Delta \dot{V}_E / \Delta$[Lactate] change of only one third of that in normal subjects. This, however, was in mildly affected patients. In severely affected patients one would anticipate an even smaller reduction in lactate levels and consequently a smaller decrease in exercise in ventilation. Most studies other than that of Casaburi *et al* have treated patients with moderate to severe disease.[49] In many patients the average FEV_1 is lower, generally about 1 litre, and in some cases less than that. Similar results in a more severely affected group of patients would be helpful before these exercise recommendations could be generalised.[56]

Exercise training to tolerance

Exercise testing and training directed at manipulation of blood lactate levels involve complex measurements and should be contrasted with the more unstructured approach of exercising to tolerance, an approach which has been used in a large number of studies.[49] These studies, despite the fact that they have not necessarily documented reductions in lactate levels, have shown that even severely obstructed patients (some with extreme hypercapnia[57]) can be exercised safely and show impressive gains in submaximal exercise endurance. This is particularly striking in the study of Niederman *et al*[58] who showed the greatest percentage improvement in those patients with the lowest FEV_1 values and low pretraining exercise endurances. In that study the training was done without emphasis on intensity, patients being allowed to choose their own exercise level. Exercise sessions were conducted three times a week for two hours for a total of nine weeks. During each session the time was divided among cycling, treadmill walking, and lifting weights. The most impressive gains were in cycle endurance which increased from 129·5 to 726·1 W/min. Similar results were obtained by Holle *et al*[59] who showed large increases in treadmill endurance.

In two recent studies large gains in endurance were achieved, although high intensity training was used and patients were encouraged to reach maximal levels of ventilation during training.[60 61] In the former study patients were initially separated into two groups based on whether an anaerobic threshold was reached. In those unable to reach an anaerobic threshold training was performed at the maximal work load achieved on the treadmill. In the patients who passed the anaerobic threshold, training intensity was initially aimed at the threshold level itself. In both groups intensity and duration were increased as tolerated. Of interest was the finding that these patients could train at exercise ventilations close to or even exceeding the maximum level reached on initial testing. In contrast to the work of Casaburi *et al*[40] both groups showed significant and comparable improvements in endurance on the treadmill. The investigators were quick to point out that this does not mean that a high intensity training regimen is therefore desirable for patients with COPD. In fact, in comparison with the previously described study,[53] gains in endurance were similar. Clearly both approaches are successful in the moderate to severely affected patient; there does not appear to be an intrinsic benefit in demanding that training be performed at almost maximal ventilatory capacity. High intensity exercise may also be disadvantageous because of the higher risk of injury and because the discomfort of extreme exercise may reduce compliance with exercise programmes.[62] These findings are summarised in Table 2.1.

Upper limb exercise training

The impact of upper extremity exercise has been discussed (see Respiratory muscle dysfunction). Ries and coworkers[63] performed a randomised study which compared a control group with two groups who used two different forms of upper arm training. Testing was done by means of cycle ergometry and unsupported arm exercise. In addition, three tests of activities of daily living were used, namely, dishwashing, dusting a blackboard, and placing grocery items on shelves. Training was performed for at least six weeks and showed that, although the patients who underwent the upper extremity training improved their performance on an arm cycle ergometer, they did not improve performance in arm activities of daily living. The specificity of limb training is emphasised by the findings of Lake et al[64] who randomised patients to one of three groups. The first group was a control group who received no training; the second group received upper limb training only; and the third group performed combined upper and lower limb training. Upper limb training included cycle ergometry with varying resistances, throwing a ball against a wall with the arms above the horizontal, passing a bean bag over the head, and arm exercise with ropes and pulleys. Lower limb exercise was tested by cycle ergometry and a six minute walk distance. Training was continued for one hour, three times a week, for eight weeks. The results showed that limb training was limb specific. Thus it was only in the group that trained with the upper extremity that upper extremity endurance increased, whereas walk distance improved in the lower limb trained group. The combination trained group showed

Table 2.1 Exercise training in COPD

	Casaburi et al[40]	Punzal et al[60]	Niederman et al[58]
No. of patients	9	57	24
FEV_1/FVC (%)	58	44	50
Intensity	High (60% of difference between anaerobic threshold and $\dot{V}o_2$max)	(1) $\dot{V}$Emax (2) At anaerobic threshold	Unstructured, laissez faire
Frequency	5/week	Daily treadmill	3/week
Duration	8 weeks inpatient 45 min cycle	Supervised 2/week × 4, then 1/week × 4 free daily unsupervised walking	9 weeks: 20 min, on cycle, treadmill, upper extremity
Test	Cycle endurance 6·6–11·4 min Anaerobic threshold ↑	Treadmill endurance 12·1–22·0 min	Cycle endurance 5·0–12·0 min 12 min walk ↑
Peak $\dot{V}o_2$ (%)	10 ↑	10 ↑	19 ↑
Psychosocial	Not measured	Breathlessness ↓ Fatigue ↓	Depression ↓ Disability ↓

improvements in both upper and lower limb endurance. A modified quality of life questionnaire was also used but only produced significant changes in the group that received combined upper and lower limb training.

Two recent studies[65][66] have confirmed the value of specific arm training. In both studies specific arm training resulted in increased arm endurance and a reduction in the metabolic cost for arm exercise. In the second study the improvements in unsupported arm activity were seen only in the group who performed unsupported exercise and not in the group who did supported arm exercise.[66] The improved endurance in conjunction with the reduced metabolic cost is indicative of improved mechanical efficiency of movement of the arms and possibly breathing muscles during arm activity.

An interesting finding of previous studies[63][64] was the lack of change in ventilatory muscle function. Before and after the upper extremity training these investigators examined ventilatory muscle endurance and neither found an improvement. Early work by Keens et al[67] in patients with cystic fibrosis suggested that upper extremity exercise may have a crossover effect and improve respiratory muscle endurance but this was not confirmed in a study of patients with COPD by Belman and Kendregan,[68] in which a group of patients who performed upper extremity cycle ergometry did not improve their ventilatory muscle endurance. Similarly, in both these studies of upper extremity training no significant change in ventilatory muscle function was found.[63][64]

Mechanisms of improvement

Improvements in exercise tolerance may be ascribed to one or more of the following factors: improved aerobic capacity, or muscle strength, or both; increased motivation; desensitisation to the sensation of dyspnoea; improved ventilatory muscle function; and improved technique of performance. Despite the multiplicity of studies performed there is, as yet, no clear consensus on the predominant mechanism of improvement.

Improved aerobic capacity

In normal subjects increased endurance has largely been ascribed to changes in the trained muscles.[69] These changes, which consist mainly of increased capillary and mitochondrial density together with increased concentrations of oxidative enzymes, occur concomitantly with training induced decreases in the exercise heart rate and constitute the major components of the aerobic training response in normal subjects.[70] Apart from the study by Casaburi et al[40] this pattern has not been observed in patients with COPD, so it is not possible to ascribe improved exercise endurance to improved aerobic performance. A striking feature of the results of exercise training in patients with COPD is the fact that, almost without exception, investigators have claimed success for their respective programmes despite the fact that training modes, intensity, and frequency have varied widely.[49] Moreover, in a study in which aerobic training effects were specifically examined by means of muscle biopsies from the trained limbs no significant improvement in oxidative enzymes was found.[71] These authors concluded that patients with COPD were unable to exercise at the threshold intensity necessary to elicit a true aerobic response.

Although the emphasis on training has concentrated on endurance activities, recent evidence supports an important role for peripheral muscle strength. A third of patients with COPD implicated muscle fatigue as the limiting factor during exercise. A subsequent randomised study evaluated the effect of a weightlifting programme in these patients.[72] The patients performed weight training three times a week for eight weeks. Both arm and leg strengthening exercises were done. The results showed an increase in cycle endurance and reduction in symptoms as assessed by a questionnaire. This study certainly reinforces the need not to neglect strength training as an important component of the training regimen.

Increased motivation

Increased motivation might easily account for the improvement seen in some studies. This could be evaluated by noting an increase in the maximal $\dot{V}\text{E}$ or heart rate. Neither of these variables has, however, increased consistently in cases where there has been an increase in endurance. In submaximal steady state exercise tests, where exercise endurance time is the measure of improvement, motivation may be a factor.

Reduction in dyspnoea

Research into the mechanisms of dyspnoea is complicated by the inherent problems with measurement of intensity of a symptom.

This topic has been reviewed recently.[73] Various scales and questionnaires are in use including the Borg scale for perceived exertion, the baseline and transitional dyspnoea indices, and the chronic respiratory disease questionnaire.[74] Moreover, techniques are available which allow measurement of quality of life. Improved measurement in these areas is essential to gauge the impact of pulmonary rehabilitation programmes in general, and exercise training in particular.

Dudley et al[47] have reviewed the psychosocial aspects of pulmonary rehabilitation and cited several studies which have found correlations between improved exercise endurance and improved feeling of well being. One study found that psychological improvement resulted from either pulmonary rehabilitation including exercises or psychotherapy alone. It has also been shown that there is a better correlation between mood and motivation and exercise endurance than between pulmonary function and exercise endurance.[75] Several studies of exercise training have shown improvements in well being and reduction in breathlessness.[49 50] In the study by Agle and coworkers[76] many of the patients also reported an improved sense of well being and decreased sensation of breathlessness after exercise training. These authors speculated that the process of graduated exercise training in the presence of trained medical personnel "inadvertently functioned as a desensitising form of behaviour therapy". They felt, therefore, that progressive exercise led to a decrease in the unrealistic fear of activity and dyspnoea. A recent study by Belman and coworkers[77] showed that four repetitive episodes of treadmill walking over 10 days at a relatively high intensity resulted in a decrease in the perceived level of breathlessness over this short period of exercise and speculated that "desensitisation" may have played a part. In a study of ventilatory muscle training[78] a control group showed significant increases in exercise after participating in the testing sequence only. This evidence has given rise to the speculation that, when patients with dyspnoea experience their symptoms in a medically controlled environment while simultaneously receiving support and encouragement, they learn to overcome the anxiety and apprehension associated with their dyspnoea. This desensitisation to dyspnoea may be a key component to improved endurance after exercise, but further investigation is necessary to prove this point.

Ventilatory muscle training

Ventilatory muscle training is not dealt with in this chapter. Its role in improving endurance is as yet unclear. A recent meta-analysis of ventilatory muscle training concluded that any effect, if present, is small and unlikely to contribute significantly to improved exercise tolerance in these patients.[79]

Improved mechanical skill

Improved skill in performance has been found in several studies including the early studies by Paez and coworkers[80] who showed that skill in treadmill walking improved with repeated attempts. Clearly, skilful performance of the task decreases both the oxygen cost and the ventilatory requirements of work, although the actual work rate is unchanged.[81] This effect constitutes training of technique and can be used to advantage in that these patients can be trained to perform specific tasks more efficiently. Although the technique of treadmill walking has been shown to improve in some studies, it is not known if this is indeed a component of improvement seen in walking other than on a treadmill.

From the large number of studies performed to date it is striking that there is no appreciable benefit on pulmonary function and gas exchange.[33 49 50] As noted above, with the singular exception of the work of Casaburi et al[40] no true aerobic training effect has been found. Even in the absence of a training effect it is impressive that there is almost universal success shown for studies of exercise training when the outcome measure is increased exercise endurance. This includes studies in which the training intensity is low. The precise mechanism responsible for the improvement is not clear, but the absence of objective cardiopulmonary improvements raises the possibility that a reduction in dyspnoea perception is important. Further research to evaluate this mechanism is required. Moreover, additional research which combines measurements of exercise as well as valid measures of breathlessness and quality of life are indicated. The transfer of improved walking endurance to increased endurance for carrying out activities to daily living also requires improved documentation.

Conclusion

Sporadic visits to the local doctor followed sometimes by changes in oral and inhaled bronchodilators and occasionally by the addition of steroids frequently does little to improve symptoms and function significantly in the disabled patient with COPD. As in other chronic diseases, the management of these patients is facilitated by a team approach in conjunction with general rehabilitation principles.[50] The rationale and practical implementation of such a programme has recently been outlined by the American Association of Cardiopulmonary Rehabilitation.[50] These are multifaceted programmes but a key component, as outlined above, is exercise training. In this brief review the various approaches available have been described. Controversy still reigns regarding the optimal modes of training and there are important differences among the several approaches. Two main groups can be delineated. One emphasises the detailed definition of the impaired physiology with therapeutic measures targeted to specific defects.[40] There is good documentation that, conversely, unstructured programmes that use treadmill and free range walking and cycling also improve endurance for walking.[59] Upper extremity training is of additional benefit. Programmes with as little as three sessions per week of 1–2 hours of low intensity activity have achieved success so we know that simple programmes can be helpful. Moreover, without the necessity for complex testing and training methods these programmes can be implemented with relatively low costs. Future investigations to examine the relationship between improved exercise capacity for walking and arm exercise on the one hand, and the ease of performance of activities of daily living on the other, will help to reinforce the effectiveness of exercise programmes.

1 Barach AL, Bickerman HA, Beck G. Advances in the treatment of non tuberculosis pulmonary disease. *Bull NY Acad Med* 1964;**1134**:28–36.
2 Gallagher CG. Exercise and chronic obstructive pulmonary disease. *Med Clin North Am* 1990;**74**:619–41.
3 Olopade CO, Beck KC, Viggiano RW, Staats BA. Exercise limitation and pulmonary rehabilitation in chronic obstructive pulmonary disease. *Mayo Clin Proc* 1992;**67**:144–57.
4 Grimby G, Stiksa J. Flow–volume curves and breathing patterns during exercise in patients with obstructed lung disease. *Scand J Clin Lab Invest* 1970;**25**: 303–13.
5 Younes M. Load responses, dyspnea, and respiratory failure. *Chest* 1990;**97**: 59–68S.
6 Regnis JA, Alison JA, Henke KG, Donnelly PM, Bye PTP. Changes in end-expiratory lung volume during exercise in cystic fibrosis relate to severity of lung disease. *Am Rev Respir Dis* 1991;**144**:507–12.
7 Stubbing DG, Pengelly LD, Morse JLC, Jones NL. Pulmonary mechanics during exercise in subjects with chronic airflow obstruction. *J Appl Physiol* 1980; **49**:511–5.

8 Babb TG, Viggiano R, Hurley B, Staats B, Rodarte JR. Effect of mild-to-moderate airflow limitation on exercise capacity. *J Appl Physiol* 1991;**70**:223–30.
9 O'Donnell DE, Sanii R, Younes M. Improvement in exercise endurance in patients with chronic airflow limitation using continuous positive airway pressure. *Am Rev Respir Dis* 1988;**138**:1510–4.
10 Petrof BJ, Calderini E, Gottfried SB. Effect of CPAP on respiratory effort and dyspnea during exercise in severe COPD. *J Appl Physiol* 1990;**69**:179–88.
11 Dodd DS, Engel L. Chest wall mechanics during exercise in patients with severe chronic air-flow obstruction. *Am Rev Respir Dis* 1984;**129**:33–8.
12 Johnson BD, Reddan WG, Seow KC, Dempsey JA. Mechanical constraints on exercise hyperpnea in a fit aging population. *Am Rev Respir Dis* 1991;**143**:968–77.
13 Spiro SG. Exercise testing in clinical medicine. *Br J Dis Chest* 1977;**71**:145–72.
14 Dillard TA. Prediction of ventilation at maximal exercise in patients with chronic airflow limitation. *Chest* 1987;**92**:195–6.
15 Dillard TA, Piantadosi S, Rajagopal KR. Prediction of ventilation at maximal exercise in chronic air-flow obstruction. *Am Rev Respir Dis* 1985;**132**:230–5.
16 Tobin MJ. Respiratory muscles in disease. *Clin Chest Med* 1988;**9**:263–86.
17 Similowski T, Sheng Y, Gauther AP, Macklem PT, Bellemare F. Contractile properties of the human diaphragm during chronic hyperinflation. *N Engl J Med* 1991;**325**:917–23.
18 Rochester DF. The Diaphragm in COPD: better than expected, but not good enough. *N Engl J Med* 1991;**325**:961–2.
19 Celli BR, Rassulo J, Make BJ. Dyssynchronous breathing during arm but not leg exercise in patients with chronic airflow obstruction. *N Engl J Med* 1986;**314**:1485–90.
20 Criner GJ, Celli BR. Effect of unsupported arm exercise on ventilatory muscle recruitment in patients with severe chronic airflow obstruction. *Am Rev Respir Dis* 1988;**138**:856–61.
21 Pardy RL, Rivington RN, Despas PJ, Macklem PT. The effects of inspiratory muscle training on exercise performance in chronic airflow limitation. *Am Rev Respir Dis* 1981;**123**:426–33.
22 Younes M. Determinants of thoracic excursions during exercise. In: Whipp BJ, Wasserman K (eds), *Exercise: pulmonary physiology and pathophysiology*. New York: Marcel Dekker, 1992:1–65.
23 Tobin MJ, Perez W, Guenther SM. Does rib cage-abdominal paradox signify respiratory muscle fatigue? *J Appl Physiol* 1987;**63**:851–60.
24 Johnson BD, Saupe KW, Dempsey JA. Mechanical constraints on exercise hyperpnea in endurance athletes. *J Appl Physiol* 1992;**73**:874–86.
25 Rochester DF. Respiratory muscle weakness, pattern of breathing, and CO_2 retention in chronic obstructive pulmonary disease (Editorial). *Am Rev Respir Dis* 1991;**143**:901–3.
26 Owens GR, Rogers RM, Pennock BE. The diffusing capacity as a predictor of arterial oxygen desaturation during exercise in patients with chronic obstructive pulmonary disease. *N Engl J Med* 1984;**310**:1218–21.
27 Dantzker DR, D'Alonzo GE. The effect of exercise on pulmonary gas exchange in patients with severe chronic obstructive pulmonary disease. *Am Rev Respir Dis* 1986;**134**:1135–9.
28 Barbera JA, Roca J, Ramirez J, Wagner PD, Ussetti P, Rodriguez-Roisin R. Gas exchange during exercise in mild chronic obstructive pulmonary disease. *Am Rev Respir Dis* 1991;**144**:520–5.
29 Wasserman K, Whipp BJ. *Principles of exercise testing and interpretation*. Philadelphia: Lea and Febiger, 1987.
30 Wilkinson M, Ranghorn CA, Heath D, Barer G, Howard PA. A pathophysiological study of 10 cases of hypoxic cor pulmonale. *Q J Med* 1988;**66**:65–85.

31 Matthay RA, Wiedemann HP. Cardiovascular pulmonary interaction in chronic obstructive pulmonary disease with special reference to the pathogenesis and management of cor pulmonale. *Med Clin North Am* 1990;**74**:571–618.
32 Nery LE, Wasserman K, French W. Contrasting cardiovascular and respiratory responses to exercise in mitral valve and chronic obstructive pulmonary diseases. *Chest* 1983;**83**:446–53.
33 Belman MJ. Exercise training in pulmonary rehabilitation. *Clin Chest Med* 1986; **7**:585–98.
34 Beaver WL, Wasserman K, Whipp BJ. Bicarbonate buffering of lactic acid generated during exercise. *J Appl Physiol* 1986;**60**:472–8.
35 Wasserman K, Beaver WL. Anaerobic threshold and respiratory gas exchange during exercise. *J Appl Physiol* 1973;**35**:236–43.
36 Beaver WL, Whipp BJ. A new method for detecting anaerobic threshold by gas exchange. *J Appl Physiol* 1986;**60**:2020–7.
37 Davis JA. Anaerobic threshold: review of the concept and directions for future research. *Med Sci Sports Exerc* 1985;**17**:6–18.
38 Brooks GA. Anaerobic threshold: review of the concept and directions for future research. *Med Sci Sports Exerc* 1985;**17**:22–31.
39 Sue DY, Wasserman K, Moricca RB, Casaburi R. Metabolic acidosis during exercise in patients with chronic obstructive pulmonary disease. *Chest* 1988;**94**: 931–8.
40 Casaburi R, Patessio A, Ioli F, Zanaboni S, Donner CF, Wasserman K. Reductions in exercise lactic acidosis and ventilation as a result of exercise training in patients with obstructive lung [see comments]. *Am Rev Respir Dis* 1991;**143**:9–18.
41 Belman MJ, Mittman C. Ventilatory muscle training improves exercise capacity in chronic obstructive pulmonary disease patients. *Am Rev Respir Dis* 1980;**121**: 273–80.
42 Belman MJ, Epstein L, Doornbos D, Elashoff J, Koerner SK, Mohsenifar Z. Reliability and validity of non-invasive detection of the anaerobic threshold in patients with chronic obstructive pulmonary disease. *Chest* 1992;**102**:1028–34.
43 Killian KJ, LeBlanc P, Martin DH, Summers E, Jones NL, Campbell EJM. Exercise capacity and ventilatory, circulatory, and symptom limitation in patients with chronic airflow limitation. *Am Rev Respir Dis* 1992;**146**:935–40.
44 Lewis MI, Belman MJ. Nutritional supplementation in ambulatory patients with chronic obstructive pulmonary disease. *Am Rev Respir Dis* 1987;**135**: 1062–7.
45 Mahler DA, Harver A. A factor analysis of dyspnea ratings, respiratory muscle strength, and lung function in patients with chronic obstructive pulmonary disease. *Am Rev Respir Dis* 1992;**145**:467–70.
46 Mahler DA, O'Connor GT. Impact of dyspnea and physiologic function on general health status in patients with chronic obstructive pulmonary disease. *Chest* 1992;**102**:395–401.
47 Dudley DL, Glaser EM, Jorganson PN. Psychosocial concomitants to rehabilitation in chronic obstructive pulmonary disease. *Chest* 1980;**77**:413–20.
48 O'Donnell DE, Webb KA. Breathlessness in patients with severe chronic airflow limitation: physiologic correlations. *Chest* 1992;**102**:824–31.
49 Ries AL. Position paper of the American Association of Cardiovascular and Pulmonary Rehabilitation. Scientific basis of pulmonary rehabilitation. *J Cardiopulmonary Rehabil* 1990;**10**:418–41.
50 Connors G, Hilling L. *Guidelines for pulmonary rehabilitation programs.* Champaign, IL: Human Kinetics, American Association of Cardiopulmonary Rehabilitation, 1992.
51 Toshima MT, Kaplan RM, Ries AL. Experimental evaluation of rehabilitation in chronic obstructive pulmonary disease: short term effects on exercise endurance and health status. *Health Psychol* 1990;**9**:237–52.

52 Cockcroft AE, Berry G. Randomised controlled trial of rehabilitation in chronic respiratory disability. *Thorax* 1981;**36**:200–3.
53 McGavin CR, Gupta SP, Lloyd EL, McHardy GJR. Physical rehabilitation for the chronic bronchitic: results of a controlled trial of exercises in the home. *Thorax* 1977;**32**:307–11.
54 Carter R, Coast JR, Idell S. Exercise training in patients with chronic obstructive pulmonary disease. *Med Sci Sports Exerc* 1992;**24**:281–91.
55 Casaburi R, Wasseman K. Exercise training in pulmonary rehabilitation. *N Engl J Med* 1986;**314**:1509–11.
56 Belman MJ, Mohsenifar Z. Reductions in exercise lactic acidosis and ventilation as a result of exercise training in patients with obstructive lung disease. *Am Rev Respir Dis* 1991;**144**:1220–1.
57 Foster S, Thomas HM. Pulmonary rehabilitation in COPD patients with elevated Pco_2. *Am Rev Respir Dis* 1988;**138**:1519–23.
58 Niederman MS, Clemente PH, Fein AM, *et al*. Benefits of a multidisciplinary pulmonary rehabilitation program. Improvements are independent of lung function. *Chest* 1991;**99**:798–804.
59 Holle RHO, Schoene RB. Increased muscle efficiency and sustained benefit in an outpatient community hospital based pulmonary rehabilitation program. *Chest* 1988;**94**:1161–8.
60 Punzal PA, Ries AL, Kaplan RM, Prewitt LM. Maximum intensity exercise training in patients with chronic obstructive pulmonary disease. *Chest* 1991;**100**:618–23.
61 Carter R, Nicotra B, Clark L, *et al*. Exercise conditioning in the rehabilitation of patients with chronic obstructive pulmonary disease. *Arch Phys Med Rehabil* 1988;**69**:118–22.
62 Belman MJ, Gaesser GA. Exercise training below and above the lactate threshold in the elderly. *Med Sci Sports Exerc* 1991;**23**:562–8.
63 Ries AL, Ellis B, Hawkins RW. Upper extremity exercise training in chronic obstructive pulmonary disease. *Chest* 1988;**93**:688–92.
64 Lake FR, Henderson K, Briffa T, Openshaw J, Musk AW. Upper-limb and lower-limb exercise training in patients with chronic airflow obstruction. *Chest* 1990;**97**:1077–82.
65 Couser JI, Martinez FJ, Celli BR. Pulmonary rehabilitation that includes arm exercise reduced metabolic and ventilatory requirements for simple arm elevation. *Chest* 1993;**103**:37–41.
66 Martinez FJ, Vogel PD, Dupont DN, Stanopoulos I, Gray A, Beamis JF. Supported arm exercise vs unsupported arm exercise in the rehabilitation of patients with severer chronic airflow obstruction. *Chest* 1993;**103**:1397–402.
67 Keens TG, Krastins IRB, Wanamaker EM, Levison H, Crozier DN, Bryan AC. Ventilatory muscle endurance training in normal subjects and patients with cystic fibrosis. *Am Rev Respir Dis* 1977;**116**:853–60.
68 Belman MJ, Kendregan BK. Physical training fails to improve ventilatory muscle endurance in patients with chronic obstructive pulmonary. *Chest* 1982;**81**:440–3.
69 Holloszy JO, Coyle EF. Adaptations of skeletal muscle to endurance exercise and their metabolic consequences. *J Appl Physiol* 1984;**56**:831–8.
70 Clausen JP. Effect of physical training on cardiovascular adjustments to exercise in man. *Physiol Rev* 1977;**57**:779–815.
71 Belman MJ, Kendregan BK. Exercise training fails to increase skeletal muscle enzymes in subjects with chronic obstructive pulmonary disease. *Am Rev Respir Dis* 1981;**123**:256–61.
72 Simpson K, Killian K, McCartney N, Stubbing DG, Jones NL. Randomised controlled trial of weightlifting exercise in patients with chronic airflow limitation. *Thorax* 1992;**47**:70–5.
73 Mahler DA, Harver A. Clinical measurement of dyspnea. In: Mahler DA (ed), *Dyspnea*. Mount Kisco, New York: Futura, 1990:75.

43

74 Guyatt GH, Chambers LW. A measure of quality of life for clinical trials in chronic lung disease. *Thorax* 1987;**42**:773–8.
75 Morgan AD, Peck DF, Buchanan DR. Effects of attitudes and beliefs on exercise tolerance in chronic bronchitis. *BMJ* 1983;**286**:171–3.
76 Agle DP, Baum GL, Chester EH. Multi-discipline treatment of chronic pulmonary insufficiency: functional status at one year follow-up. In: Johnston RF, ed. *Pulmonary medicine*. A Hahnemann Symposium. New York: Grune and Stratton, 1973:355.
77 Belman MJ, Brooks LR, Ross DJ, Mohsenifar Z. Variability of breathlessness measurement in patients with chronic obstructive pulmonary disease. *Chest* 1991;**99**:566–71.
78 Levine S, Weiser P, Gillen J. Evaluation of a ventilatory muscle endurance training program in the rehabilitation of patients with COPD. *Am Rev Respir Dis* 1986;**133**:400–6.
79 Smith K, Cook D, Guyatt GH, Madhavan J, Oxman AD. Respiratory muscle training in chronic airflow limitation: a meta-analysis. *Am Rev Respir Dis* 1992;**145**:533–9.
80 Paez PN, Phillipson EA, Masangkay M, Sproule BJ. The basis of training patients with emphysema. *Am Rev Respir Dis* 1967;**95**:944–53.
81 Lustig FM, Haas A, Castillo R. Clinical and rehabilitation regime in patients with COPD. *Arch Phys Med Rehabil* 1972;**53**:315–22.

3 Ventilatory muscle training

ROGER S GOLDSTEIN

Although in recent years ventilatory muscle function has received considerable attention, the role of ventilatory muscle training within the context of the management of patients with altered ventilatory function remains unclear. It is likely that ventilatory muscles will function less well—that is, will be unable to maintain their required or expected force[1] if their rate of energy consumption exceeds that of their energy supply. The energy demands are influenced by the work of breathing and the integrity of the contractile apparatus,[2-4] whereas the energy supply is determined by the force and timing of muscle contraction and by the delivery of oxygen to the tissues.[5] Training of the ventilatory muscles must follow the basic principles of training for any striated muscle with regard to the intensity and duration of the stimulus, the specificity of training, and the reversibility of training. It is equally important to evaluate the outcome of training with appropriate end points. Although there are many conditions in which the ventilatory muscles are involved, most published reports have been of healthy volunteers or subjects with chronic airflow limitation. This chapter will discuss the standard methods used for testing and training of the ventilatory muscles, the rationale for such training, and the results of training programmes. It will end with conclusions for the clinician as to whether it is appropriate to include ventilatory muscle training as part of the management of those with respiratory conditions.

Muscle strength

As in any striated muscle, the force of contraction will be determined by:

1 The length of the muscle (length–tension relationship)
2 Whether the contraction is associated with shortening (force–velocity relationship)
3 The strength and frequency of stimulation (force–frequency relationship)
4 The integrity of the contractile apparatus.[6]

The length of the respiratory muscles varies with lung volume. Inspiratory muscle contractile force is greatest between functional residual capacity (FRC) and residual volume (RV), and expiratory muscle contractile force is greatest at total lung capacity (TLC). Although a bedside evaluation of a short sniff or a strong cough will reflect a subject's respiratory muscle strength, the standardised laboratory method of evaluating strength is that described by Black and Hyatt[7] in which the subject is encouraged to make maximal efforts against a closed airway. More invasive measurements include ballooned catheter assessments of oesophageal (pleural) and gastric (abdominal) pressures and their difference, the transdiaphragmatic pressure (P_{DI}). The P_{DI} recorded during a sniff from FRC provides an accurate and reproducible measure of inspiratory muscle strength[8] and oesophagheal pressure recorded during a cough reliably reflects expiratory muscle strength.[9] Recently there has been considerable interest in bilateral simultaneous transcutaneous phrenic nerve stimulation in the assessment of diaphragmatic strength. Not only is this method relatively painless, but it allows for an accurate and reproducible measure of muscle strength without requiring a maximal effort from the subject. The amplitude of the shock is monitored from the muscle mass action potential (M wave) recorded with surface electrodes. A non-invasive measure of diaphragmatic contractility can be achieved by measuring mouth pressure against an occluded airway during phrenic nerve twitch stimulation. With the glottis open and the airway closed at the mouth, mouth pressure is a good estimate of the overall pressure change on the pleural surface.[10 11]

Muscle endurance

Ventilatory muscle endurance will be determined by the composition of muscle fibre types, the adequacy of the blood

46

supply, and the integrity of the contractile apparatus.[6] It will also be influenced by the force and duration of contraction and the velocity of shortening during the contraction. Because the force of contraction is expressed in relation to its maximal value, muscle strength will have an important influence on endurance.

Tests of endurance

Hyperpnoea

The laboratory evaluation of endurance has included measurements of sustained ventilation and sustained pressure. The simplest is the maximum voluntary ventilation (MVV), a brief period (12 or 15 seconds) during which the subject is encouraged to sustain maximum ventilation with no extrinsic ventilatory load. The test reflects voluntary neural drive, airway resistance, and respiratory muscle strength.[12 13] In 1968 Tenney and Reese[14] studied isocapnic hyperpnoea and reported that the logarithm of endurance time varied linearly (negative slope) with the percentage of maximal breathing capacity (20 second MVV). They also reported that estimates of power of breathing against endurance time were consistent with a simple model in which energy is derived from a fixed finite store and from a steady supply. The rate of supply was estimated to be adequate to sustain ventilation at 55% of maximal breathing capacity. Leith and Bradley[15] later evaluated the influence of ventilatory muscle endurance using sustained isocapnic hyperpnoea and noted that the sustained ventilatory capacity, when plotted against endurance time, became asymptotic at about 80% of MVV. Studies among healthy volunteers, subjects with chronic obstructive pulmonary disease, and those with cystic fibrosis have reported that their maximum sustained ventilatory capacity for 15 minutes was between 60% and 100% of MVV.[16-18]

Resistive loading

Measurements of endurance based on the time for which subjects could overcome alinear inspiratory resistive loads have become popular following a classic study by Roussos and Macklem.[19] In this study healthy volunteers were invited to breathe to exhaustion against an alinear inspiratory resistance at a given, predetermined, transdiaphragmatic pressure which was measured with two balloons and displayed to the subject on an oscilloscope. At FRC the P_{DI} that could be generated indefinitely was about 40% of the $P_{DI}max$,

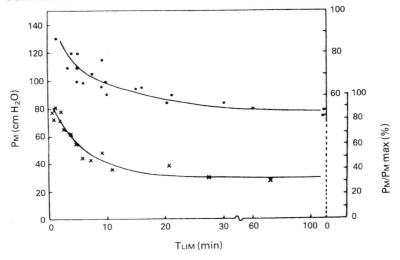

Figure 3.1   Effect of lung volume on endurance time (TLIM) in minutes. Left ordinate: mouth pressure (PM); right upper ordinate: mouth pressure as percentage of maximum (PM/PMmax) at functional residual capacity (●); right lower ordinate: PM/PMmax at functional residual capacity $+ 0.5$ inspiratory capacity (x). Note difference in asymptotic value of PM/PMmax at the two lung volumes. (Reproduced with permission from Roussos *et al.*[20])

with contraction and relaxation times being relatively equal. In a subsequent study these authors showed that, if the same inspiratory load applied at FRC was applied at a higher lung volume, the inspiratory muscle endurance time was reduced (Figure 3.1).[20]

Given that the diaphragm contracts during inspiration it should tire more rapidly if, at any given tension, the ratio of inspiratory time to the duration of the breathing cycle (TI/TTOT) is increased. Bellemare and Grassino[21 22] have pointed out that the duty cycle is an important component of inspiratory muscle endurance. For the diaphragm they proposed a tension–time index (TTDI) which incorporated both the pressure (PDI/PDImax) and the duty cycle (TI/TTOT). The TTDI in healthy volunteers becomes critical at about 0.15. This critical index of work is similar to the tensions known to cause limitation of blood flow in other skeletal muscles. In an open chest animal model[23] it was shown that blood flow was limited beyond a TTDI of 0.2. The physiological implication of this finding is that, if the diaphragm is obligated to exceed its critical tension, its ability to perform work will be limited by its

$\dot{V}o_2$ during relaxation when blood flow is restored and it may fail. This explanation was also suggested by Tenney and Reese[14] to explain the limitation during sustained hyperventilation at greater than 50% of maximal breathing capacity. In measurements of endurance that use alinear inspiratory resistive loads, the pattern of breathing should be standardised. If this is the case, highly accurate and reproducible measures of inspiratory muscle endurance can be made.

Threshold loading

In 1982 Nickerson and Keens[24] devised a method for measuring ventilatory muscle endurance as the sustainable inspiratory pressure which is the highest pressure a subject can generate in each breath for 10 minutes. A weighted plunger was used as an inspiratory valve which ensured that a minimum pressure was generated with each breath (Figure 3.2). In 15 healthy volunteers aged between 5 and 75 years the mean (SE) sustainable inspiratory pressure was 82 cm H_2O or 68% (3%) of their maximum inspiratory pressure. This method allows for reproducible measurements of ventilatory muscle endurance. Clanton et al[25] have shown that both inspiratory flow rate and duty cycle will influence the sustainable inspiratory pressure and therefore these variables should be standardised. Chen and Kuo[26] tested 160 healthy volunteers using this technique and reported that:

1 Endurance was greater in men who were physically active than in those who were sedentary
2 It was higher in men than in women
3 It decreased with age.

Martyn et al[27] described an incremental test of ventilatory muscle performance in which threshold loads were progressively increased at two minute intervals. Subjects began with a low load and continued to breathe until they could no longer inspire. The authors concluded that this two minute incremental loading test was a simple assessment of ventilatory muscle performance. The practical significance of such a test remains to be explored.

Repeated maximal static contractions

A more recent approach to the measurement of respiratory muscle endurance described by Gandevia et al involves repeated maximal contractions against a closed airway.[28] With this technique

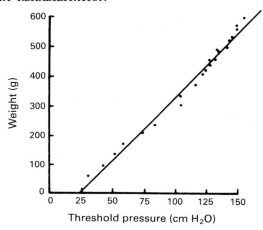

Figure 3.2 Relationship between weight on plunger and threshold mouth pressure. $r = 0.99$; $p < 0.0001$. (Reproduced with permission from Nickerson and Keens.[24])

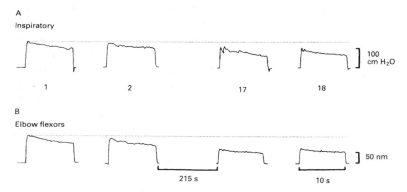

Figure 3.3 Records from a typical study in a control subject. Repeated maximal static contractions of (A) the inspiratory muscles at functional residual capacity and (B) the elbow flexor. The contractions lasted 10 seconds with rest intervals of five seconds (duty cycle of 67%). Note the decline in peak and average sustained force was less for the inspiratory muscles than for the elbow flexors. (Reproduced with permission from Newell et al.[29])

it has been suggested that the inspiratory muscles recover more rapidly from fatigue than do the expiratory muscles or limb muscles (Figure 3.3). This technique has the advantage of allowing respiratory muscles to be compared with limb muscles under similar

50

Table 3.1   Properties of muscle fibre types

Characteristic	Fibre type		
	I	IIA	IIB
Twitch type	Slow	Fast	Fast
Colour	Intermediate	Red	White
Myosin ATPase activity	Low	High	High
Glycolytic capacity	Low	Intermediate	High
Oxidative capacity	High	High	Low
Mitochondrial density	High	High	Low
Endurance capacity	Excellent	Good	Poor

Reproduced from Rochester[6] with permission.

circumstances and its use has been reported both in healthy volunteers and in subjects with respiratory disease.[28 29]

Histochemical composition

It has become clear that the performance of the respiratory muscles is linked to their histochemical composition (Table 3.1). This property of all skeletal muscle is reflected in its fibre types. Generally type I fibres have a high oxidative capacity and a relatively low concentration of glycolytic enzymes. They are activated by smaller motor neurons recruited early during the orderly recruitment of motor units and, although they produce low levels of force relative to their cross sectional area, they are fatigue resistant. The time from the onset of contraction to peak tension is slow and they are referred to as slow twitch fibres. Type IIA muscle fibres are intermediate in oxidative capacity, enzyme concentration, and fatigue resistance. Type IIB muscle fibres are low in oxidative capacity and have a high concentration of glycolytic enzymes. They are activated by larger motor neurons recruited later during the orderly recruitment of motor units and they fatigue rapidly. The time from the onset of contraction to peak tension is fast and they are referred to as fast twitch fibres. In the diaphragm of normal adults there are about 55% type I fibres whereas pre-term infants, who may be prone to muscle dysfunction, have less than 10%.[30]

Rationale for training

Initial studies of ventilatory muscle training have been on healthy volunteers.[15 24 25] When healthy volunteers are encouraged to

Table 3.2   Diseases sometimes associated with respiratory muscle weakness

Neurological diseases	Quadriplegia Myasthenia gravis Botulism Poliomyelitis Guillain–Barré syndrome
Muscle diseases	Myopathy (for example, steroids) Specific muscle enzyme deficiencies
Connective tissue diseases	Polymyositis Dermatomyositis Systemic lupus erythematosus
Endocrine disorders	Thyrotoxicosis Cushing's disease
Metabolic disorders	Hypophosphataemia Hypocalcaemia, hypomagnesaemia Metabolic alkalosis

breathe to exhaustion[31] at levels of ventilation close to their MVV there are measurable changes in the pressure–frequency relationship of the diaphragm, the ratio of high to low frequency power of the diaphragmatic electromyograph, and in the PDImax. These observations suggest that ventilatory endurance at high levels of ventilation may be limited by ventilatory muscle fatigue. Such levels of ventilation are rarely encountered in day to day activities and therefore ventilatory muscle training is unlikely to be of value among healthy individuals. When ventilatory muscle training was applied to healthy volunteers in peak athletic condition ($\dot{V}o_2$max >60 ml/kg per min) it did not influence maximum oxygen uptake or endurance cycling at 90% of maximal power output.[32]

In contrast, there are several diseases in which the ventilatory muscles may influence gas exchange, the level of physical activity, or the sensation of dyspnoea (Table 3.2). Such limitations unquestionably influence the quality of life and, if muscle training were to result in a useful functional improvement, it would be indicated as part of the management of these conditions (see chapter 11).

Methods of ventilatory muscle training

As in testing, the training regimens have focused on repeated maximal inspiratory and expiratory efforts against a closed airway

Table 3.3   Effect of hyperpnoeic training on ventilatory muscles

Reference	No. of subjects	Endurance Duration (min)	Frequency (weeks)	Course (weeks)	Response* (%)	Better than control subjects?
Leith and Bradley[15]	4 normal	20–30	5	5	19	Yes
Keens et al[16]	4 normal	25	5	4	22	—
	4 with CF	25	5	4	55	Yes
Belman and Mittman[18]	10 with COPD	30	5	6	33	—
Levine et al[17]	15 with COPD	15	5	6	41	Yes
Reis and Moser[33]	5 with COPD	30	5	6	16	No

* Increased in maximum sustained ventilatory capacity. COPD = chronic obstructive pulmonary disease. CF = cystic fibrosis.
Reproduced with permission from Belman.[34]

for strength training and isocapnic hyperpnoea, resistive and pressure threshold loads for endurance training. Isocapnic hyperpnoea has been shown to improve test function among healthy volunteers and subjects with cystic fibrosis and chronic obstructive pulmonary disease (Table 3.3). Leith and Bradley[15] have shown that, after five weeks of ventilatory muscle training, subjects trained for strength increased their strength by 55% whereas those who trained for endurance increased their maximum sustained ventilatory capacity from 81% to 96% of their MVV (Table 3.4). This very well designed study emphasised the importance of the specificity of training and the importance of the stimulus being sufficiently high to effect training. The programme consisted of training for five days a week for five weeks. Strength trainers performed repeated maximal static inspiratory and expiratory manoeuvres against obstructed airways, and endurance trainers performed isocapnic hyperpnoea to exhaustion at levels of ventilation equivalent to 50% MVV.

Alinear resistances have also been applied to the inspiratory muscles for training. The response to training has been measured either as the maximum tolerable resistance or as the time during which a given load may be sustained. Pardy et al[35] used a simple home programme in which subjects inspired for 30 minutes per day

Table 3.4   Ventilatory muscle response to training

	Control group	Strength trainers	Endurance trainers
Strength at FRC			
PEmax	4 (6)	57 (9)*	10 (9)
PImax	−2 (6)	54 (16)*	9 (13)
Lung volumes			
TLC	0·7 (1·3)	4·6 (1·4)*	1·9 (0·8)
VC	−0·3 (2·2)	3·6 (0·8)	3·1 (1·2)
Sustained ventilatory capacity (% MVV)	4·5 (1·5)	3·8 (1·5)	15·5 (5·0)*
MVV at 15 seconds	0·8 (4·0)	2·0 (0·7)	14 (4·7)*

FRC, functional residual capacity; PEmax, maximum expiratory pressure; PImax, maximum inspiratory pressure; TLC, total lung capacity; VC, vital capacity; MVV, maximum voluntary ventilation. Values are change in percentage (SE). *Statistically significant change (independent t test).
Reproduced with permission from Leith and Bradley.[15]

(in two 15 min sessions) against their critical inspiratory resistance while watching television or reading a book. At the end of two months of training the critical resistance that could be tolerated by the subject had increased. Many training programmes have incorporated this approach. Unfortunately, subjects often change their breathing strategy to one of slow, deep inspirations in order to tolerate more easily the inspiratory resistance. This strategy almost certainly reduces the inspiratory load to a level below that necessary to induce training. It is therefore essential that the breathing pattern is controlled during training. Belman and Shadmehr[36] overcame this issue during resistive ventilatory muscle training by using a single orifice resistance together with a target feedback device. The feedback device regulated breathing frequency, duty cycle, and mean pressure. Two other studies have reported the influence of resistive training during which there was some control over the pattern of breathing and the mean mouth pressure achieved.[37 38]

Clanton et al[39] showed the effectiveness of the threshold loading technique in training four healthy volunteers for half an hour each day over 10 weeks. The mean (SD) maximal inspiratory pressure increased by 50 (9) cm H_2O and the endurance time for a load set at 65% of the initial maximal inspiratory pressure increased by six minutes. Both Clanton et al[39] and Goldstein et al[40] controlled for duty cycle, frequency, and tidal volume (Figure 3.4).

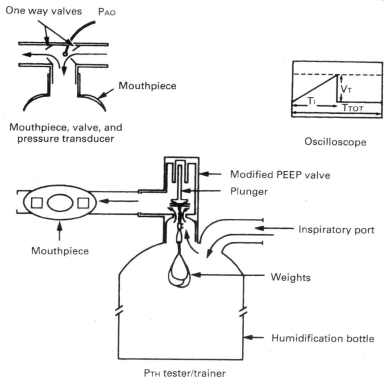

One way valves   PAO

Mouthpiece

Mouthpiece, valve, and
pressure transducer

Oscilloscope

Modified PEEP valve

Plunger

Mouthpiece

Inspiratory port

Weights

Humidification bottle

PTH tester/trainer

Figure 3.4   Diagram of PTH tester/trainer with details of mouthpiece and information shown to subject during testing. PAO, pressure at the airway opening (expressed as mean mouth pressure); PEEP, positive end expiratory pressure. (Reproduced with permission from Goldstein.[40])

Response to training

Normal skeletal muscles will adapt to training provided that the appropriate stimulus is applied.[41-44] The basic principles of training are:

1 For muscle fibres to change structure and function they must be stressed (overloaded) above a critical threshold
2 Training is specific for the stimulus—that is, strength training will increase fibre size (muscle hypertrophy) whereas endurance training will increase oxidative enzymes and mitochondrial density, myoglobin content, and capillary density

3 Training is reversible and the effects will be reduced (deconditioning) if the training ceases.

Ventilatory muscles will undergo extensive metabolic adaptation to chronically increased respiratory loads, presumably to optimise muscle performance.[42 44 46] It appears, however, that training does not produce any major shifts in the proportion of slow twitch and fast twitch fibres in skeletal muscle although there are no longitudinal studies that have encompassed a large enough sample and included all of the techniques used in the identification of fibre type interconversion.[47] Muscle will also adapt to maximise its length–tension characteristics by altering the number of its sarcomeres.[48-51] This process of adaptability of skeletal muscle may have an important bearing on the indications for training those patients with chronic respiratory disease. Keens et al[16] noted that subjects with cystic fibrosis had a 36% higher ventilatory muscle endurance than did healthy volunteers and suggested that a process of adaptation to the chronic stress of breathing against high inspiratory loads had occurred. Similowski et al[52] evaluated the contractile properties of the human diaphragm during chronic hyperinflation and concluded that, for the same lung volume, the function of the diaphragm was as good as that measured in healthy volunteers.

Chronic obstructive pulmonary disease

There are good theoretical reasons to think that subjects with chronic obstructive pulmonary disease may be expected to develop ventilatory muscle dysfunction as their work and energy cost of breathing are substantially increased, whereas their capacity to endure such work may be diminished by mechanical and other influences.[34 53] The main mechanical change is that of hyperinflation which shortens the inspiratory muscles and puts them in a disadvantageous position on their length–tension curve. Hyperinflation results in a significant decrease in the size of the zone of apposition between the costal fibres of the diaphragm and the rib cage (see Figure 2.2 on page 21).[54] The increased airway resistance results in an increased inspiratory load with each breath so the work of breathing is increased at rest and during exercise. COPD also influences the size and mass of the diaphragm as part of the generalised weight loss that patients often experience. This weight loss probably relates to the increased caloric requirements in subjects in whom intake is inadequate. Another influence of ventilatory muscle function in patients with COPD may be that of drugs such as steroids which could further compromise muscle function. These influences on muscle function may be closely linked to dyspnoea and to limitations in exercise performance.

A superb review of the physiological and clinical aspects on training of the respiratory muscles has recently been published by Grassino.[55] Given that maximum inspiratory pressure and PDImax are reduced, there may be merit for strength training. As it has been recognised that the sensation of dyspnoea is related to the percentage of the maximum inspiratory pressure developed with each breath,[56] it is possible that strengthening the inspiratory muscles may lessen dyspnoea. Strengthening of expiratory muscles may assist with clearance of secretions. Endurance training might result in an increased capacity for higher levels of ventilation (such as in physical exercise) or for sudden increases in resistive load (such as in infectious exacerbations). There is some preliminary evidence that inspiratory resistive training may assist those with chronic respiratory failure in being weaned from mechanical ventilation by providing brief periods of fatiguing exertion alternating with periods of complete rest.[57] Subjects with COPD (bronchitis, emphysema, asthma, cystic fibrosis, bronchiectasis) could, at least in theory, benefit from training.

Results of training programmes

A very large number of studies have evaluated the influence of ventilatory muscle training and the reader is referred to two recent reviews for details of several published studies.[34 58] In summary, it appears that subjects can be trained to improve their performance as measured by a particular test of endurance which is specific to the training modality. The evidence that such training results in functionally useful changes remains equivocal. Smith *et al*[59] recently reviewed 73 articles from a computerised bibliographical database and identified 17 relevant randomised trials of ventilatory muscle training in chronic airflow limitation. The study quality was assessed and descriptive information concerning the study populations, interventions, and outcome measurements was extracted. The authors then combined effect sizes across studies (the difference between treatment and control groups divided by the pooled standard deviation of the outcome measure). The criteria for methodological quality are shown in Table 3.5. A primary analysis of these results showed that only MVV was associated with a significant p value for the effect size. A secondary analysis was undertaken in which studies were included only if ventilatory muscle training was associated with control of the breathing pattern. These studies were compared with those in which breathing pattern had not been controlled (Table 3.6). The authors concluded that respiratory muscle strength and endurance will improve, but with no associated alterations in functional exercise capacity or laboratory measurements of exercise capacity.

Although most of the above studies have involved subjects with chronic bronchitis and emphysema, ventilatory muscle function has also been improved in subjects with cystic fibrosis.[16 60] Keens

Table 3.5   Criteria for methodological quality*

Sample
   Random or consecutive sample (5)
   Arbitrary sample (or cannot tell) (0)

Similarity of groups
   Number of following variable in which groups were comparable: age, gender, forced expiratory volume, maximum inspiratory pressures, walk test distance (0–5)

Cointervention
   Number of following criteria met: comparable frequency of visits, comparable medication changes, comparable number of intercurrent illnesses (5 for 3/3; 3 for 1/3; 0 for 0/3)

Sham or masking
   Sham or masking undertaken (5)
   No sham or masking (0)

Compliance
   Training was hospital supervised (5)
   Home programme with reporting diary and patients periodically (4)
   Home programme with either diary or periodic review (3)
   Compliance not measured or cannot tell (0)

Observer masking
   Observers masked as to treatment groups (5)
   Not masked or cannot tell (0)

Standardised testing
   Encouragement standardised (5)
   Not standardised or cannot tell (0)

Follow up
   90–100% follow up (5)
   80–89% follow up (3)
   <80% subjects accounted for (1)
   Cannot tell (0)

* Numbers in parentheses indicate number of points in summary score.
Reproduced with permission from Smith et al.[59]

Table 3.6 Sensitivity analysis of resistance studies with flow rates controlled versus those with flow rates not controlled

Variable/condition	No. of studies	Effect size (standard deviation units)	Effect size (natural units)	p	Homogeneity p	p value*
Respiratory muscle strength (PImax), controlled flow rate	5	0·51	8·2 cm	0·01	0·92	
Respiratory muscle strength (PImax), uncontrolled flow rate	6	−0·09	−1·8 cm	0·57	0·23	0·02
Respiratory muscle endurance, controlled flow rate	4	0·41	10·3 l/min	0·06	0·93	
Respiratory muscle endurance, uncontrolled flow rate	3	−0·08	−14·6 l/min	0·67	0·23	0·09
Laboratory exercise capacity, controlled flow rate	2	−0·002	−0·02 ml/kg per min	0·99	0·10	
Laboratory exercise capacity, uncontrolled flow rate	5	−0·17	−1·57 ml/kg per min	0·10	0·09	0·30
Functional exercise capacity, controlled flow rate	3	0·30	88·9 m†	0·22	0·75	
Functional exercise capacity, uncontrolled flow rate	4	0·07	18·4 m	0·71	0·05	0·45
Functional status, controlled flow rate	2	0·65	1·87‡	0·02	0·004	
Functional status, uncontrolled flow rate	3	−0·13	−0·70	0·49	0·92	0·02

PImax, maximal inspiratory pressure. * On difference in effect size between controlled and uncontrolled studies; †12 minute walking test distance; ‡ dyspnoea rate of chronic respiratory questionnaire in which 0·5 is minimal important difference.
Reproduced with permission from Smith et al.[59]

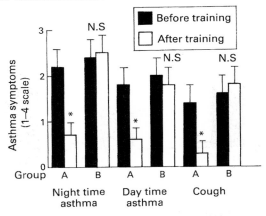

Figure 3.5 Mean (SE) diary card data for asthma symptoms judged by the patients on a scale of 0 = no symptoms to 4 = very severe symptoms before and during the last two weeks of training. Group A received inspiratory muscle training and group B received sham training. *$p < 0.05$; NS, not significant. (Reproduced with permission from Weiner *et al.*[61])

et al[16] were able to induce changes in ventilatory muscle endurance of equivalent magnitude to that of endurance training in seven subjects who participated in a four week physical activity training programme consisting of 1·5 hours per day of swimming and canoeing. A recent report by Weiner *et al*[61] described the results of inspiratory muscle training among asthmatic subjects: 15 subjects (group A) received inspiratory muscle training and 15 (group B) were assigned to sham training in a double blind trial. Unfortunately the pattern of breathing during testing and training was not controlled. Subjects reported improvements in several indices of asthma in association with improvements in strength and endurance (Figure 3.5) including a reduction in the amount of inhaled β_2 agonists.

Outstanding issues

The above studies of ventilatory muscle training raise a number of interesting issues. First, the use of whole body exercise to evaluate ventilatory muscle function may not be appropriate as it involves many other muscle groups unrelated to breathing. The evidence that physical exercise is associated with ventilatory muscle dysfunction rests, in fact, on a few uncontrolled studies in a small

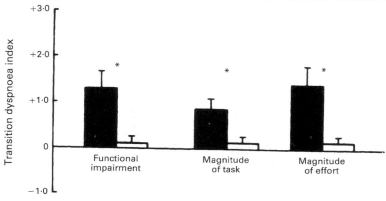

Figure 3.6 Mean scores for each category of the transition dyspnoea index for both experimental (solid bars) and control (open bars) subjects. Bar represents one standard error. Asterisk indicates significant difference between experimental and control conditions. (Reproduced with permission from Harver et al.[38])

number of subjects.[58 62] In these subjects exercise was associated with measured changes in the ratio of the high to low frequencies in the power spectrum of the diaphragmatic electromyogram.

Second, only a few studies have explored measurements of dyspnoea and of quality of life before and after ventilatory muscle training. Patessio et al[63] reported that there was a reduction in dyspnoea at each inspiratory load in trained subjects but not in a placebo group and concluded that training against an inspiratory resistance decreased the sensation of breathlessness in association with an increase in inspiratory muscle strength and endurance. Dekhuijzen et al[37] found no differences in psychometric measures of anxiety, depression, and physical complaints between those who completed a respiratory rehabilitation programme with inspiratory muscle training and control subjects who completed only a respiratory rehabilitation programme. Harver et al[38] reported that study subjects showed a decrease in dyspnoea after eight weeks of training which was reflected in an improvement in scores of the transition dyspnoea index (Figure 3.6); control subjects did not. There is therefore a need for better quantification of the sensation of dyspnoea before and after ventilatory muscle training.

Third, the role of expiratory muscle training has been relatively unexplored. During isocapnic hyperpnoea expiratory muscle training almost certainly occurs, but during inspiratory resistive loading the role of the expiratory muscles is less clear. Recent studies among healthy volunteers have confirmed that during exercise and during inspiratory resistive loading the expiratory muscles are increasingly activated and there may be changes to the power spectrum of their electromyogram.[64-66] Whether there is a specific role for expiratory muscle training remains to be clarified.

Finally, although harder to evaluate than strength or endurance training, improvements in the coordination of respiratory muscle function may be of benefit to some patients. Following whole body exercise, improvements in performance, in the absence of cardiovascular or skeletal muscle training, may relate to improvements in neuromuscular coordination and the efficiency of breathing. Pursed lip breathing, which is learned naturally by some patients, may minimise lung hyperinflation. Emphasis on diaphragmatic and abdominal breathing may reduce dyspnoea. The role of training coordination needs to be defined as it might be complementary to whole body exercise and to specific training of the ventilatory muscles for strength or endurance.

Conclusion

The subject of ventilatory muscle training is a fascinating study of the application of the principles of training any striated muscle to the muscles of the ventilatory system. Training for strength and endurance has been achieved in healthy subjects and in those with chronic airflow limitation but only a few studies are available that describe the influence of training in other conditions. When training has occurred the evidence that it resulted in changes that were functionally useful is, at best, equivocal. Training against resistive loads or pressure threshold loads has generally focused on the muscles of inspiration and there is little information on the effect of training the expiratory muscles. Natural adaptations of the muscles of respiration might mitigate against the need for training by maximising their function against chronically increased loads. Whole body exercise is probably an inappropriate outcome measure. Studies of gas exchange, quality of life, and dyspnoea are still needed. The design of training programmes must take into consideration an adequate training stimulus, in terms of both intensity and duration, and must control for the pattern of breathing. Ventilatory muscle training is not recommended at present by this author as part of the routine management of those with chronic ventilatory conditions. There is, however, considerable potential for research that might identify the appropriate population for training, the best modality of training, and the role of training within the context of other modalities of rehabilitation.

Acknowledgment

Supported by West Park Hospital Foundation and the Network of Centres of Excellence—Respiratory Health.

1 Edwards RHT. Physiological analysis of skeletal muscle weakness and fatigue. *Clin Sci Mol Med* 1978;**54**:463–70.
2 Macklem PT. Respiratory muscles: the vital pump. *Chest* 1980;**78**:753–8.
3 Rochester DF, Arora NS. Respiratory muscle failure. *Med Clin North Am* 1983; **67**:573–97.
4 Roussos CS. The failing respiratory pump. *Lung* 1982;**160**:59–84.
5 Bellemare F, Grassino A. Force reserve of the diaphragm in patients with chronic obstructive pulmonary disease. *J Appl Physiol* 1983;**55**:8–15.
6 Rochester DF. Tests of respiratory muscle function. *Clin Chest Med* 1988;**9**: 249–61.
7 Black LF, Hyatt RE. Maximal respiratory pressures: normal values and relationship to age and sex. *Am Rev Respir Dis* 1969;**99**:696.
8 Miller MJ, Moxham J, Green M. The maximal sniff in the assessment of diaphragm function in man. *Clin Sci* 1985;**69**:91–7.
9 Arora NS, Galt J. Cough dynamics during progressive expiratory muscle weakness in healthy curarized subjects. *J Appl Physiol* 1981;**51**:494–8.
10 Bellemare F, Bigland-Ritchie B. Assessment of human diaphragm strength and activation using phrenic nerve stimulation. *Respir Physiol* 1984;**58**:263–77.
11 Yan S, Gauthier A, Similowski T, Macklem P, Bellemare F. Evaluation of human diaphragm contractility using mouth pressure twitches. *Am Rev Respir Dis* 1992;**145**:1064–9.
12 Lavietes MH, Clifford E, Silverstein D, Stier F, Reichman LB. Relationship of static respiratory muscle pressure and maximum voluntary ventilation in normal subjects. *Respiration* 1979;**38**:121–6.
13 Aldrich TK, Arora NS, Rochester DF. The influence of airway obstruction and respiratory muscle strength on maximal voluntary ventilation in lung disease. *Am Rev Respir Dis* 1982;**126**:195–9.
14 Tenney SM, Reese RE. The ability to sustain great breathing efforts. *Respir Physiol* 1968;**5**:187–201.
15 Leith DE, Bradley M. Ventilatory muscle strength and endurance training. *J Appl Physiol* 1976;**41**:508–16.
16 Keens TG, Krastins IRB, Wanamaker EM, *et al.* Ventilatory muscle endurance training in normal subjects and patients with cystic fibrosis. *Am Rev Respir Dis* 1977;**116**:853–60.
17 Levine S, Weiser P, Gillen J. Evaluation of a ventilatory muscle endurance training program in the rehabilitation of patients with chronic obstructive pulmonary disease. *Am Rev Respir Dis* 1986;**133**:400–6.

18 Belman MJ, Mittman C. Ventilatory muscle training improves exercise capacity in COPD. *Am Rev Respir Dis* 1980;**121**:273–80.
19 Roussos CS, Macklem PT. Diaphragmatic fatigue in man. *J Appl Physiol* 1977; **43**:189–97.
20 Roussos CS, Fixley M, Gross D, Macklem PT. Fatigue of inspiratory muscles and their synergic behaviour. *J Appl Physiol* 1979;**46**:897–904.
21 Bellemare F, Grassino A. Evaluation of human diaphragm fatigue. *J Appl Physiol* 1982;**53**:1196–206.
22 Bellemare F, Grassino A. Effect of pressure and timing of contraction on human diaphragm fatigue. *J Appl Physiol* 1982;**53**:1190–5.
23 Bellemare F, Wright D, Lavigne CM, Grassino A. Effect of tension and timing of contraction on the blood flow of the diaphragm. *J Appl Physiol* 1983;**54**: 1597–606.
24 Nickerson BG, Keens TG. Measuring ventilatory muscle endurance in humans as sustainable inspiratory pressure. *J Appl Physiol* 1982;**52**:768–72.
25 Clanton TL, Dixon GF, Drake J, Gadek JE. Effects of breathing pattern on inspiratory muscle endurance in humans. *J Appl Physiol* 1985;**59**:1834–41.
26 Chen HI, Kuo CS. Relationship between respiratory muscle function and age, sex and other factors. *J Appl Physiol* 1989;**66**:943–8.
27 Martyn JB, Moreno RH, Pare PD, Pardy RL. Measurement of inspiratory muscle performance with incremental threshold loading. *Am Rev Respir Dis* 1987;**135**:919–23.
28 Gandevia SC, McKenzie DK, Neering IR. Endurance properties of respiratory and limb muscles. *Respir Physiol* 1983;**53**:47–61.
29 Newell SZ, McKenzie DK, Gandevia SC. Inspiratory and skeletal muscle strength and endurance and diaphragmatic activation in patients with chronic airflow limitation. *Thorax* 1989;**44**:903–12.
30 Keens TG, Bryan AC, Levison H, Ianuzzo CD. Developmental pattern of muscle fibre types in human ventilatory muscles. *J Appl Physiol* 1978;**44**:909–13.
31 Bai TR, Rabinovitch BR, Pardy RL. Near maximal voluntary hyperpnea and ventilatory muscle function. *J Appl Physiol* 1984;**57**:1742–8.
32 Fairbarn MS, Coutts KC, Pardy RL, McKenzie DC. Improved respiratory muscle endurance of highly trained cyclists and the effects on maximal exercise performance. *J Sports Med* 1991;**12**:66–70.
33 Reis AL, Moser KM. Comparison of isocapnic hyperventilation and walking exercise training in pulmonary rehabilitation. *Chest* 1986;**90**:285–9.
34 Belman MJ. Ventilatory muscle training and unloading. In: Casaburi R, Petty TL (eds), *Principles and practice of pulmonary rehabilitation*. Philadelphia: Saunders, 1993.
35 Pardy RL, Rivington N, Despas PJ, Macklem PT. The effects of respiratory muscle training on exercise performance in chronic airflow limitation. *Am Rev Respir Dis* 1981;**123**:426–33.
36 Belman MJ, Shadmehr R. Targeted resistive ventilatory muscle training in chronic obstructive pulmonary disease. *J Appl Physiol* 1988;**65**:2726–35.
37 Dekhuijzen PNR, Folgering HTM, Van Herwaarden CLA. Target flow inspiratory muscle training during pulmonary rehabilitation in patients with COPD. *Chest* 1991;**99**:128–33.
38 Harver A, Mahler DA. Daubenspeck JA. Targeted inspiratory muscle training improves respiratory muscle function and reduces dyspnea in patients with chronic obstructive pulmonary disease. *Ann Intern Med* 1989;**111**:117–24.
39 Clanton TL, Dixon G, Drake J, Gadek JE. Inspiratory muscle conditioning using a threshold loading device. *Chest* 1985;**87**:62–6.
40 Goldstein RS, De Rosie J, Long S, Dolmage T, Avendano MA. Applicability of a threshold loading device for inspiratory muscle testing and training in patients with COPD. *Chest* 1989;**96**:564–71.

41 Faulkner JA. Structural and functional adaptations of skeletal muscle. In: Roussos C, Macklem PT (eds), *Thorax* New York: Marcel Dekker, 1985: 1324–52.
42 Holloszy JO. Adaptations of muscular tissue to training. *Prog Cardiovasc Dis* 1976;**18**:445–58.
43 Keens TG, Chen V, Patel P, *et al.* Cellular adaptations of the ventilatory muscles to a chronic increased respiratory load. *J Appl Physiol* 1978;**44**:905–8.
44 Leiberman DA, Maxwell LC, Faulkner JA. Adaptation of guinea pig diaphragm muscle to aging and endurance training. *Am J Physiol* 1972;**222**:556–60.
45 Tarasiuk A, Scharf SM, Miller MJ. Effect of chronic resistive loading on inspiratory muscles in rats. *J Appl Physiol* 1991;**70**:216–22.
46 Farkas GA, Roussos CS. Adaptability of the hamster diaphragm to exercise and/or emphysema. *J Appl Physiol* 1982;**53**:1263–72.
47 Saltin B, Gollnick PD. Skeletal muscle adaptability: significance for metabolism and performance. In: Peachey LD, Adrian RH, Geiger SR (eds), *Handbook of physiology: skeletal muscle*. Bethesda, Maryland: American Physiological Society, 1983:555–631.
48 Dudley GA, Abraham WM, Terjung RL. Influence of exercise intensity and duration on biochemical adaptations in skeletal muscle. *J Appl Physiol* 1982; **53**:844–50.
49 Kelsen SG, Wolanski T, Supinski GS, Roessmann U. The effect of elastase-induced emphysema on diaphragmatic muscle structure in hamsters. *Am Rev Respir Dis* 1983;**127**:330–4.
50 Supinski GS, Kelsen SG. Effect of elastase induced emphysema on the force generating ability of the diaphragm. *J Clin Invest* 1982;**70**:978–88.
51 Farkas GA, Roussos CD. Diaphragm in emphysematous hamsters: sarcomere adaptability. *J Appl Physiol* 1983;**54**:1635–40.
52 Similowski T, Sheng Yan MD, Gauthier AP, Macklem PT, Bellemare F. Contractile properties of the human diaphragm during chronic hyperinflation. *N Engl J Med* 1991;**325**:917–23.
53 Rochester DF, Arora NS, Braun NMT, Goldberg SK. The respiratory muscles in chronic obstructive pulmonary disease (COPD). *Bull Eur Physiopathol Respir* 1979;**15**:951–75.
54 Tobin MJ. Respiratory muscles in disease. *Clin Chest Med* 1988;**9**:263–86.
55 Grassino A. Inspiratory muscle training in COPD patients. *Eur Respir J* 1989; **2**:581–6s.
56 Killian KJ, Campbell EJM. Dyspnea. In: Roussos C, Macklem P (eds), *The Thorax—Part B*. New York; Marcel Dekker, 1985:787–828.
57 Aldrich TK. The patient at risk of ventilator dependency. *Eur Respir J* 1989;**2**: 645–51s.
58 Pardy RL, Reid WD, Belman MJ. Respiratory muscle training. *Clin Chest Med* 1988;**9**:287–96.
59 Smith K, Cook D, Guyatt GH, Madhavan J, Oxman AD. Respiratory muscle training in chronic airflow limitation: a meta-analysis. *Am Rev Respir Dis* 1992; **145**:533–9.
60 Asher MI, Pardy PL, Coates AL, Thomas E, Macklem PT. The effects of inspiratory muscle training in patients with cystic fibrosis. *Am Rev Respir Dis* 1982;**126**:855–9.
61 Weiner P, Azgad Y, Ganam R, Weiner M. Inspiratory muscle training in patients with bronchial asthma. *Chest* 1992;**102**:1357–61.
62 Grassino A, Gross D, Macklem PT, Roussos CS, Zagelbaum G. Inspiratory muscle fatigue as a factor limiting exercise. *Bull Eur Physiopathol Respir* 1979; **15**:105–11.
63 Patessio A, Rampulla C, Fracchia C, *et al.* Relationship between perception of breathlessness and inspiratory resistive loading: report on a clinical trial. *Eur Respir J* 1989;**2**:587–91s.

64 Abbrecht PH, Rajagopal KR, Kyle RR. Expiratory muscle recruitment during inspiratory flow-resistive loading and exercise. *Am Rev Respir Dis* 1991;**144**: 113–20.
65 Suzuki S, Susuki, J, Okubo T. Expiratory muscle fatigue in normal subjects. *J Appl Physiol* 1991;**70**:2632–90.
66 Suzuki S, Suzuki J, Ishii T, Akahori T, Okubo T. Relationship of respiratory effort sensation to expiratory muscle fatigue during expiratory threshold loading. *Am Rev Respir Dis* 1992;**145**:461–6.

4 Pharmacological interventions in COPD

MICHAEL G PEARSON

Chronic obstructive pulmonary disease (COPD) is a slowly progressive disorder in which patients progress from normality to a state of severe dyspnoea and respiratory failure over a variable period of between 20 and 50 years. The defining lesion is airflow limitation in all cases, but this can be the result of varying degrees of emphysema (high compliance and large airway collapse during expiration), chronic bronchitis (with mucosal gland hypertrophy and small airway disease), and chronic asthma (which has become refractory to asthma therapy). COPD differs from moderate asthma physiologically in that the airflow limitation cannot be fully reversed by use of bronchodilator or anti-inflammatory drugs, and also clinically in that the history is usually one of gradual progressive decline without periods of intervening "wellness". The natural history of COPD is also different in that it begins in a well person and over many years evolves sequentially through mild and moderate phases before becoming severe disease. This is a one way process. Thus, therapy is directed at slowing progression and relieving (but not curing) pulmonary deficits, while also treating acute intermittent infective exacerbations. The clinical stages of COPD are summarised in Table 4.1; as can be seen from this, it is convenient to divide COPD into its mild, moderate, and severe phases when considering the therapeutic options.

At any stage of COPD the most important first step of prevention in a smoking patient is to get him or her to stop. The rate of decline of lung function accelerates with continuing years of smoking and in spite of available treatments.[1 2] In mild disease smoking cessation is likely to prevent the patient ever reaching the moderate or

67

Table 4.1

	Clinical state	Results of measurements
Mild	"Smoker's cough" but no breathlessness No abnormal signs	FEV_1 between 60 and 79% of predicted. FEV_1/VC ratio and other indices of expiratory flow mildly reduced
Moderate	Breathlessness ($\pm$wheeze) on exertion, cough ($\pm$sputum) and some abnormal signs	FEV_1 of 41–59% of predicted with often increases in FRC and reductions in DLCO. Some patients hypoxic but not hypercapnic
Severe	Breathless on any exertion. Wheeze, cough prominent. Clinical hyperinflation usual plus cyanosis and polycythaemia in some	FEV_1<40% predicted, with marked hyperinflation. DLCO variable but often low. Hypoxia usual and hypercapnia in some

Modified from Calverly PMA, Pride NB (eds), *Chronic obstructive pulmonary disease*, London: Chapman & Hall, 1994:317.
FEV_1, forced expiratory volume in 1 second; VC, vital capacity; DLCO, carbon monoxide diffusing capacity.

severe stages,[3] whereas in severe disease it reduces the number of exacerbations and, for example, allows the benefits of long term oxygen therapy to be realised.[4] This important non-pharmacological intervention must be neither forgotten nor overlooked when considering any of the therapeutic options described below.

Relieving pulmonary impairment: bronchodilators

In the relief of bronchopulmonary impairment, bronchodilators are the most important medication and so a good deal of this chapter is devoted to their study. Alternative drugs are discussed at the end.

Bronchodilators act to relax smooth muscle in the bronchial and bronchiolar walls. In asthma administration of bronchodilator can have dramatic effects both on the measure of flow limitation and often the patients' symptoms. In COPD this is only one of the mechanisms that limit airflow and often only a minor component. The permanent damage within the lungs[5]—the fixed small airway disease, the reduced lung elasticity and increased compliance, plus airway collapsibility during expiration—cannot be influenced by drugs and the response is therefore often very limited. It is debatable whether the airway smooth muscle tone is actually increased in COPD. In many cases it is probable that the bronchodilator is simply relaxing the normal resting level of bronchial muscle tone, resulting in very small changes in measurable lung function change.

More than half the patients with severe COPD (forced expiratory volume at one second or FEV_1 of about 1 litre) will show some response in FEV_1 after treatment with a bronchodilator, but in only a very small number will the response be as large as 0·5 l.[6 7] These drugs may, however, act by methods other than by improving the FEV_1. Hay and colleagues[8] showed that the anticholinergic drug oxitropium bromide could produce reductions in breathlessness both before and after a six minute walking test. The reduced breathlessness was associated with being able to walk further and applied whether or not there was an FEV_1 response. Spence et al[9] from the same group showed that, in a larger cohort, similar functional benefit could be related to changes in the lung mechanics and in particular to reduced air trapping as reflected by the functional residual capacity (FRC). A different index of air trapping (the difference between total lung capacity measured with body plethysmography and that measured with helium dilution methods) correlated with the improvement in exercise ability in a study of 33 patients given oral theophyllines for eight weeks.[10] This interesting observation has not as yet been replicated in other laboratories.

As most of the changes induced by bronchodilators in COPD are small, it is remarkably difficult to define clear end points against which to assess the effectiveness of a particular drug and thus whether it is worth prescribing. For example, if in a large sample the size of the FEV_1 change is plotted on a frequency chart, there is a continuum of response from no change (or a small fall) to substantial increase. The reproducibility of the FEV_1 measurement is such that changes of less than 200 ml are within the error of the measurement[11] and both American[12] and European[13] guidelines now stipulate that a response can only be considered significant if it exceeds 200 ml. Such arbitrary cut off figures are useful when analysing group data in studies, but unhelpful when trying to assess, for example, the individual who has shown an increase in FEV_1 of 190 ml after a drug. Similar problems apply to all the other assessments of response including six minute and 12 minute walks, breathlessness scores, symptom scores, and quality of life measures. Thus the clinician is left to make an overall judgment, which often is decided by whether the patient "feels that the drug helps" and by taking into account the risks and benefits of treatment.

Types of bronchodilator and routes of administration

There are three classes of bronchodilator which may be useful in COPD: β agonists and anticholinergics are available as metered dose inhalers, dry powder inhalers, nebulised solutions, and tablets; theophyllines are available as slow release tablet preparations. In asthma, the inhaled route has been shown to produce better results with fewer side effects than oral preparations and so it is always to be preferred.[14] Lung deposition of inhaled preparations becomes progressively less effective as airflow obstruction increases,[15] with greater proportions of drug being deposited in the trachea and main bronchi. Despite this, COPD patients have also been shown to respond better or as well after inhaled β agonists with less side effects than after the oral equivalent.[16] Dose–response studies have shown that most COPD patients who are able to respond will do so at doses equivalent to between two and eight actuations of a metered dose inhaler.[17] Side effects of oral medication, including theophyllines (see below), mean that oral drugs are relegated to second line therapy.

Thus, the first choice of bronchodilator at any stage of COPD is between an inhaled β agonist (salbutamol 200 μg or terbutaline 500 μg) or an anticholinergic (ipratropium bromide 40 μg or oxitropium 200 μg) via either a metered dose aerosol or a dry powder inhaler. Whether β agonists are better bronchodilator drugs than anticholinergic drugs is a controversial issue with strong commercial overtones. β agonists have a faster onset of action and thus may be preferred by patients using the bronchodilator for relief of acute symptoms but the anticholinergic may have a longer duration of action.[18] In the form of metered dose or dry powder inhalers, both drug types have an excellent safety record so that they can be safely prescribed to any COPD patient. They are both relatively cheap and most COPD patients report some degree of acute symptomatic benefit, so almost all COPD patients with symptoms should have a "reliever" inhaler. Such comment does not, however, apply to higher dose preparations (see below).

The long acting inhaled β agonists (salmeterol and formoterol) have not been systematically studied in COPD. They might be expected to produce the same small increases in FEV_1 as short acting drugs, but whether this is as clinically useful as the fast onset, short acting drugs remains speculative, and at the time being they cannot be recommended for routine use—at least until confirmatory data are produced. A similar argument can be advanced for the slow release, oral β agonist preparations (slow release salbutamol and bambuterol) which have the added therapeutic disadvantage of being oral preparations. All these preparations may eventually prove to have a better safety profile than the oral theophyllines, but, based on current knowledge, theophyllines (when used carefully) have the advantage of a proven track record.

Factors to consider in selecting a bronchodilator

In asthma the UK guidelines recommend a β agonist as first line bronchodilator therapy, reserving anticholinergic inhalers until step 4 of the five treatment steps.[19] In COPD the β agonists are very widely used and there is good evidence of their efficacy as symptom relievers,[8] although the relative advantages of β agonists over anticholinergic drugs are unclear. A number of studies have compared the spirometric efficacy of the different drugs and most have concluded that they are equipotent in COPD.[20 21] There is some evidence that individual patients may respond better to one than the other. Most of these studies have been either single dose or of very short duration, so it is not known if the results equate with a long term effect. Nisar et al[22] showed that, in 100 patients with severe COPD, one third responded to single doses of both drugs, one sixth to β agonist alone, one sixth to anticholinergic alone, and one third to neither, with FEV_1 responses of similar magnitude. The IPPB (intermittent positive pressure breathing) trial[8] demonstrated that single dose testing can produce very variable results—thus one third of patients testing positive on one occasion will be negative when re-tested on a second occasion and vice versa. The overall magnitude and frequency of responses do not, however, change over time. The largest and longest bronchodilator study used the anticholinergic ipratropium bromide on 5887 patients in a parallel group, double blind, five year study as part of the American Lung Health Study[22] which looked at the effects of smoking cessation and bronchodilator use on FEV_1 decline. It showed that ipratropium improved the FEV_1 by an average of 26 ml and that the improvement was maintained over the five years. Ipratropium did not affect the rate of decline of lung function and, once it was stopped at the end of the study, the effect was lost. In other words, the bronchodilator provided a temporary increase in FEV_1 without affecting the underlying disease process. In contrast, smoking cessation led to an initial improvement in FEV_1 and a reduced rate of decline there-after—thereby confirming the original work of Fletcher nearly 20 years earlier.[23] The newer anticholinergic oxitropium 200 μg has been reported to be better than ipratropium 40 μg in COPD,[24] although another study[25] has suggested that at the higher dose of 80 μg the two are equipotent. More data are needed on this issue.

Theophyllines are available in a number of slow release, oral tablet formulations. The slow release mechanism means that their onset is delayed, so they are of no value for relieving acute dyspnoea, although a proportion of COPD patients like the mild prolonged bronchodilatation and find tablets easier to take than inhalers. The major limitation is the high incidence of minor side effects, particularly gastric symptoms, and the smaller risk of serious problems such as epileptic fits and cardiac dysrhythmias.[26 27] Monitoring and control of serum levels are possible, but not always easy because absorption varies with the different products[28] and metabolism is influenced by a number of factors including cigarette smoking.[29] Up to 10% of patients attending emergency departments have levels in the toxic range.[30] If theophyllines are to be used, the serum levels should be checked and the dose titrated to the therapeutic range—there are a number of computer algorithms to help with this process.[31] If the problems of dosage and toxicity can be overcome then there is good evidence that theophyllines will increase the mean FEV_1 in group studies by up to 20%,[10 32 33] a result comparable to the inhaled bronchodilators.[34]

Not all patients will show a spirometric response, and many will report benefits in exercise tolerance or just in "well being". The FEV_1 is measurable and of concern to the physician, but the patient is more likely to be concerned with changes in exercise ability and breathlessness. A substantial improvement in FEV_1 is likely to be associated with a corresponding beneficial effect on the patient's exercise ability and feeling of well being. Two studies,[8 9] already referred to, noted better performance and/or less breathlessness even in those without an improved FEV_1 in response to an anticholinergic. Other studies confirm that such changes apply to the other classes of bronchodilators, theophyllines,[10 35 36] and β agonists.[37 38] It is probable that these benefits are related to a reduction in hyperinflation and an associated improvement in the mechanics of the lung, diaphragm, and chest wall muscles. Whether the contractility of the diaphragm and respiratory muscles is directly affected by, for example, theophylline[39] remains a debatable point.[40]

Combinations of bronchodilators

Combining a β agonist and an anticholinergic produces a better short term response than either agent used singly,[20 38 41 42] and this may be true for combinations of either agent with theophyllines.[43] It is difficult to be certain of the exact relationship between single agents and combinations because the doses used vary between studies as do the patient selection criteria. The studies have been reviewed[44] and can probably be summarised best by saying that β agonists, anticholinergics, and theophyllines can all improve FEV_1 and/or produce symptomatic benefit to a roughly equal degree and combinations result in more benefit for some patients. The picture is, however, confused by the doses employed.

What dose and how often?

There remain considerable doubts concerning the optimum dosage for a given patient. The shape of the dose–response curve is contentious. Some workers have claimed that there is continued response as doses of salbutamol are increased up to 2000 μg and more by inhaler or by nebuliser,[45 46] whereas others would argue that for many patients the dose–response curve is flat beyond about 800 μg. Increasing the dose will increase the side effects (see below), but in general, as the β agonists and anticholinergic drugs have excellent safety records, physicians have not been afraid to prescribe high doses. The concerns about regular β agonist therapy in asthma[47] may also apply in COPD[48] and could be expected to be most worrying at high doses. There is still, however, a degree of disbelief about the dangers in asthma and the Dutch group have suggested, in a more recent communication,[49] that their initial views may have been incorrect. As these drugs are given to relieve acute symptoms, it is logical to prescribe them on an "as required" basis. Most physicians will prescribe a metered dose or dry powder inhaler in a standard dose as needed for symptoms. The patient will then use it as much as he or she needs to gain the most subjective benefit and many choose to take regular doses. The physician can then monitor progress with serial FEV_1 measurements and assessments of symptoms, but given the small changes occurring in most patients, and the variability of the available measurements, most patients receive these drugs in the long term on the basis of whether the patient reports that he or she "feels better" or not.

Nebulised treatment

Many patients with severe COPD have acute exacerbations and upon admission to hospital are given nebulised bronchodilators. As this has given them relief, such patients will often then ask their doctor if they can have nebulised drugs on a regular basis. Nebulisers are devices that deliver a high dose of β agonist and/or anticholinergic with no effort or coordination from the patient. The dose–response studies[45 50] show that FEV_1 may respond better to high doses and there is some evidence that tachyphylaxis does not occur,[7] so that one might expect some benefit to continue. At high doses the side effects are, however, increased and problems such as hypokalaemia[51 52] are potentially more worrying in patients with ischaemic heart disease.[53] Which patients derive benefit and, indeed, whether any long term benefits accrue from high dose treatment remain controversial. In the only double blind study comparing nebulised salbutamol with salbutamol by spacer, more patients preferred the nebuliser even when it contained the saline placebo.[54] This raises the question of whether it is the salbutamol or the humidification that is most beneficial, and there is evidence to show that saline does improve mucus clearance.[55] The following is the best advice at the moment to patients with severe disease:

1 Be fully assessed by a respiratory physician to confirm COPD
2 Try simple inhalers and a range of devices
3 If still symptomatic, have a trial of home nebuliser therapy while recording both peak expiratory flow (PEF) and symptoms
4 If mean PEF rises by more than 15% or there is clear symptomatic benefit, the nebuliser can be continued.

It is still unclear what symptom change constitutes a "clear benefit" and also whether that benefit necessarily continues over time. There is no evidence to show that use of high dose nebuliser either prolongs life or results in deleterious side effects. A major disadvantage of nebulisers is the cost of treatment. The device costs only about £100 in the United Kingdom, but taken four times daily the drugs cost £559 per annum for β agonist and £590 for anticholinergic at current UK prices.[56] Standard dose, metered dose inhalers cost less than £40. Until better documented and larger outcome studies of high dose therapy over longer periods have been done, nebulisers should be reserved for the very few who cannot gain similar benefit with conventional doses or even high doses by metered dose inhaler or dry powder inhaler.

74

What outcome

As some patients show a spirometric response, whereas others become less breathless and others simply "feel better", it is impossible to set a single outcome measure. The optimum dose has to be set by knowledge of the general properties of these drugs and the objective and subjective changes interpreted by both the physician and the patient, taking into account benefits and side effects. It is not easy to explain to patients or to other health professionals that, although a small amount of drug may help, they should not expect a greater effect from a higher dose. It is important not to judge the response in COPD by the responses observed in asthmatic patients because the disease processes are not directly comparable. This means that there is almost always good justification for prescribing standard doses of bronchodilator to all patients with moderate to severe COPD, but progressively less indications for higher doses, culminating in a very small number of patients needing high dose regular therapy by nebuliser.

Mode of delivery

About 50% of patients with asthma have difficulty using a metered dose inhaler device and the same is true in COPD, especially as most patients are elderly.[57][58] Although many more can be taught successfully to use a metered dose inhaler, there is, however, no equivalent available for COPD patients to the network of asthma nurses. Elderly patients can use the breath actuated, metered dose inhalers better.[59][60] Alternatives are the dry powder inhalers but these have the disadvantage of doubling drug costs. Nebulisers are also possible to use with elderly people, but have the disadvantage of cost and also of increased side effects because there is a high incidence of concurrent cardiac and other disease.

Inhaled steroids

In asthma there is unequivocal evidence of benefit from the use of inhaled steroids. Substantial doses can be given without serious side effects and with few drawbacks. Inhaled steroids are believed to reduce the inflammation of the airways which is the major pathological process in asthma. As COPD is also associated with airway narrowing and inhaled steroids are a very safe group of drugs, it has been tempting to use them widely. COPD is, however, the result of a number of different processes and there is no

75

evidence that, for example, steroids will have any effect on the emphysematous loss of elastin and associated alveolar destruction. There is some evidence of inflammatory change in the airways in at least some patients with COPD,[61] and a number of the patients with COPD will have reached this stage because of chronic irreversible asthma. About 20–25% of COPD patients can be shown to have a clinically significant FEV_1 response to an oral steroid trial (30 mg prednisolone for two weeks),[62] and for these steroid responsive patients there is some evidence that they have a better outcome.

Rimmington et al[63] have shown that, in a cohort of 211 patients with moderate to severe COPD, the 21% with a steroid response had significantly better five year survival, and survivors also had better lung function. Whether inhaled steroids have any effect on the rate of progression of COPD in patients non-responsive to oral steroids remains uncertain. The evidence so far derives from subanalyses of studies designed to test other hypotheses[63 64] and is insufficient to justify routine prescription of inhaled steroids in COPD. There are two major European studies in progress (EUROSCOP (European Study of Corticosteroids in Obstructive Pulmonary Disease) and ISOLDE (Inhaled Steroids in Obstructive Lung Disease in Europe)—both are unlikely to be reporting until 1998–9) and these should have sufficient power and numbers to provide clear direction on this point.

Use of drugs when diagnosing COPD

If a patient presents with airflow limitation, then regardless of severity the physician should find out how much of the deficit is reversible. About half of an unselected group of patients with moderate to severe COPD presenting to an outpatient department have a response to nebulised β agonists and, of these, just under half (21% of initial cohort) have a significant response to 30 mg oral prednisolone over two weeks.[62] If the airflow limitation can be fully reversed with either therapy then, by definition, the patient has asthma and should be treated accordingly. If there is a substantial response to the steroid, then the patient should have an inhaled steroid and also be treated in much the same way as for asthma. Some would define these patients as asthmatic even though, on initial clinical presentation, physiology, and laboratory measurements, they are indistinguishable from the non-responder

COPD patients.[62] When there is no response to steroid but a response to the bronchodilator then this seems to be of little prognostic value in deciding future treatment strategies,[65] although it may help in defining best obtainable lung function for that individual.

Managing the acute attack

Acute exacerbations are rare in mild, unusual in moderate, but common in severe COPD. An acute exacerbation of COPD is not a worsening of the underlying COPD pathology; it is the result of an additional problem, usually an infection, superimposed on already impaired lungs. Therapy should be directed towards the additional factor, while also supporting the lung function throughout the crisis. Full assessment will always include arterial blood gas measurement and prescription of an appropriate level of oxygen support (often 24% or 28%).

It is usual to treat the acute exacerbation with high dose nebulised bronchodilators and oral corticosteroids. The rationale for this approach is largely derived by extrapolation from asthma trials and there are few studies in COPD[41 50] justifying this approach. The evidence that combinations of β agonist and anticholinergic drugs are better as first line therapy than either agent alone is also rather weak, although it is common practice. Although there may be no real concern and only modest additional cost from using a combination on arrival at hospital, there is evidence that, once improvement is seen, one or other should be stopped at least in nebulised form.[67]

Clues to the presence of infection are the combination of changing sputum colour, increased breathlessness, and increased sputum volume. If all three are present it is prudent to begin empirical antibiotic treatment. Sputum culture is rarely available in time to be useful in COPD and the relationship of such cultures to the clinical picture is also not clear. The most common bacteria are *Haemophilus influenzae*, pneumococci and *Moraxella* sp., so that, for community acquired exacerbations, antibiotics such as amoxycillin or erythromycin are suitable. When patients come to hospital who have already received one or more antibiotics in primary care, co-amoxiclav is probably a better first choice;[66] if there is no marked response over the first 24 hours it would be appropriate to go higher up the antibiotic ladder with the choice being dictated by knowledge of the local bacteriological sensitivity patterns. Unless the patient is *in extremis*, the antibiotics can be given orally. Once an acute infection has been cleared there is no evidence to support the use of antibiotics prophylactically. A more pragmatic approach is to give patients a course of antibiotics for them to keep at home with instructions to start the course as soon as their sputum become "dirty". Such an approach is common but has never been scientifically validated.

Summary of treatments at each stage of the disease

Mild COPD	Need strong anti-smoking advice Few symptoms so that most will not even need a bronchodilator
Moderate COPD	Need strong anti-smoking advice Breathlessness usually sufficient to justify and get benefit from a single drug bronchodilator inhaler—unlikely to need combinations of bronchodilators Antibiotics for exacerbations A steroid trial useful diagnostically and if positive should have inhaled steroids Unlikely to require oral steroids even in exacerbations
Severe COPD	Very symptomatic and limited Will always need an inhaled bronchodilator and often will report benefit from combinations of β agonist and anticholinergic Subject to side effects—theophyllines may help An oral steroid trial can help select patient for regular inhaled steroids Acute exacerbations often severe requiring hospital care and oral steroids, antibiotics, nebulised bronchodilators, and sometimes respiratory support. Selected patients will need further long term support to maintain an acceptable quality of life

Oral steroids are often used in the acute episode, but unlike for asthma there is very little evidence to support this practice. Most British doctors will give the patient a dose of 30 mg prednisolone for 7–10 days; until a proper study is performed, this "habitual" prescribing is likely to continue.

Cough mixtures, sputum thinners, and expectorants

Cough with or without sputum is present in up to 80% of patients with moderate to severe COPD.[68] The most common cause is cigarette smoking and, if patients can be persuaded to stop smoking, then within six months 94% will have lost their cough.[69] Expectorants have no proven useful effect,[70] and have been removed from the list of prescribable medications in the United Kingdom. Bronchodilators are claimed to improve mucociliary clearance[71 72] but whether the effects are clinically useful is disputed.[73 74] Drugs that thin mucus in vitro such as N-acetylcysteine have been reported to reduce the number of exacerbations in vivo,[75] but these data have not been readily reproduced and these drugs are little used in the United Kingdom, although still popular in Europe. The newer agents which act to lyse DNA in the sputum have likewise not yet been shown to have effects that are clinically important.

Other drugs and treatments

In very severe COPD there are a number of extra problems associated with severe hypoxia and with cor pulmonale. Oxygen therapy is of proven benefit and is discussed in chapter 7 whereas cor pulmonale often requires additional active therapy with one or more of the following: diuretic, digoxin, and/or angiotensin converting enzyme inhibitor. The non-pharmacological treatments, including social support and pulmonary rehabilitation programmes, are discussed elsewhere in this book.

1 Fletcher CM, Peto R, Tinker C, Speizer FC. *The natural history of chronic bronchitis and emphysema.* Oxford: Oxford University Press, 1976.
2 Burrows B, Knudsen RJ, Camilli AE, *et al.* The horse-racing effect and predicting decline in forced expiratory volume in one second from screening spirometry. *Am Rev Respir Dis* 1987;**135**:788–93.

3 Traver GA, Cline MG, Burrows B. Predictors of mortality in COPD. *Am Rev Respir Dis* 1979;**119**:895–902.
4 Medical Research Council Working Party. Long term domiciliary oxygen therapy in chronic hypoxic cor pulmonale complicating chronic bronchitis and emphysema. *Lancet* 1981;**1**:681–6.
5 Lamb D. Pathology. In Calverly PMA, Pride NB (eds), *Chronic obstructive pulmonary disease*. London: Chapman & Hall, 1994:9–34.
6 Nisar M, Walshaw MJ, Earis JE, Pearson MG, Calverley PMA. Assessment of airway reversibility of airway obstruction in patients with chronic obstructive airways disease. *Thorax* 1990;**45**:190–4.
7 Anthonisen NR, Wright EC, and the IPPB Trial group. Bronchodilator response in chronic obstructive pulmonary disease. *Am Rev Respir Dis* 1986;**133**:814–19.
8 Hay JG, Stone P, Carter J, *et al.* Bronchodilator reversibility, exercise performance and breathlessness in stable chronic obstructive pulmonary disease. *Eur Respir J* 1992;**5**:659–64.
9 Spence DPS, Hay JG, Carter J, *et al.* Oxygen desaturation and breathlessness during corridor walking in chronic obstructive pulmonary disease. *Thorax* 1993; **48**:1145–50.
10 Chrysten H, Mulley BA, Peake MD. Dose response relation to oral theophylline in severe chronic obstructive airways disease. *BMJ* 1988;**297**:1506–10.
11 Tweedale PM, Alexander F, McHardy GJR. Short-term variability in FEV_1 and bronchodilator responsiveness in patients with chronic obstructive ventilatory defects. *Thorax* 1987;**42**:487–90.
12 American Thoracic Society. Lung function testing: Selection of reference values and interpretative strategies. *Am Rev Respir Dis* 1991;**144**:1202–8.
13 Quanjer PH. Standardised lung function tests. *Eur Respir J* 1993;**6**:53–102.
14 Tattersfield A. Asthma management and treatment. In: Brewis A, Gibson JG, Geddes DM (eds), *Respiratory Medicine*. London: Baillière Tindall, 1990: 1199–1220.
15 Pavia D, Thompson ML, Clarke SW, Shannon HS. Effect of lung function and mode of inhalation on penetration of aerosol into the human lung. *Thorax* 1977;**32**:144–97.
16 Shim CS, Williams MH. Bronchodilator response to oral aminophylline and terbutaline, aerosol sabuterol in patients with chronic obstructive pulmonary disease. *Am J Med* 1983;**75**:697–701.
17 Corris P, Neville E, Nariman S, Gibson GJ. Dose–response study of inhaled salbutamol powder in chronic airflow limitation. *Thorax* 1983;**38**:292–6.
18 Gross NJ. Ipratropium bromide. *N Engl J Med* 1988;**319**:486–94.
19 Guidelines on the Management of Asthma. *BMJ* 1993;**306**:776–82; *Thorax* 1993;**48**:S1–24.
20 Nisar M, Earis JE, Pearson MG, Calverley PMA. Acute bronchodilator trials in chronic obstructive pulmonary disease. *Am Rev Respir Dis* 1992;**146**:555–9.
21 Tashkin DP, Ashutosh K, Bleeker ER, *et al.* Comparison of the anticholinergic bronchodilator ipratropium bromide with metaproterenol in chronic obstructive pulmonary disease: a 90 day multicentre study. *Am J Med* 1986;**81**:81–90.
22 Anthonisen NR, Connett JE, Kiley JP, *et al.* The Lung Health Study: Effects of smoking intervention and the use of an inhaled anticholinergic bronchodilator on the rate of decline of FEV_1. *JAMA* 1994;**272**:1497–505.
23 Fletcher C, Peto R. The natural history of chronic airflow obstruction. *BMJ* 1977;**i**:1645–8.
24 Takishima T, Sekizawa K, Tamura G, Inoue H. Anticholinergics in treatment of COPD—site of bronchodilatation. *Clin Res Forums* 1990;**13**:49–59.
25 Peel ET, Anderson G, Cheong B, Broderick N. A comparison of oxitropium bromide and ipratropium bromide in asthma. *Eur J Respir Dis* 1984;**65**:106–8.
26 Bowton DL, Alford PT, McLees BD, *et al.* The effects of aminophylline on cerebral blood flow in patients with chronic obstructive lung disease. *Chest* 1987;**91**:874–7.

27 Levine JH, Michel JR, Guarnien T. Multifocal atrial tachycardia. A toxic effect of theophylline. *Lancet* 1985;**ii**:12–14.

28 McElnay JC, Smith GD, Helling DR. A practical guide to interactions involving theophylline kinetics. *Drug Intell Clin Pharm* 1982;**16**:533–42.

29 Powell JR, Thiercelin JF, Vozen S, *et al*. The influence of cigarette smoking and sex on theophylline disposition. *Ann Rev Respir Dis* 1977;**116**:17–23.

30 Sessler CN. Theophylline toxicity: clinical features of 116 consecutive cases. *Am J Med* 1990;**88**:567–76.

31 Chrystyn H, Mulley BA, Peake MD. The accuracy of a pharmacokinetic theophylline predictor using once daily dosing. *Br J Clin Pharmacol* 1987;**24**: 301–7.

32 Alexander MR, Dull WL, Kasik JE. Treatment of chronic obstructive pulmonary disease with orally administered theophylline. *JAMA* 1980;**244**:2286–90.

33 Jenkins PF, White JP, Jariwalla AJ, *et al*. A controlled study of slow release theophylline and aminophylline in patients with chronic bronchitis. *Br J Dis Chest* 1982;**76**:57–60.

34 Fikuk RB, Easton PA, Anthonisen NR. Responses to large doses of salbutamol and theophylline in patients with chronic obstructive pulmonary disease. *Am Rev Respir Dis* 1985;**132**:871–4.

35 Mahler DA, Matthaway A, Snyder PE, Wells CK, Loke J. Sustained release theophylline reduces dyspnoea in non-reversible obstructive airway disease. *Am Rev Respir Dis* 1985;**131**:L22–5.

36 Mulloy E, McNicholas WT. Theophylline improves gas exchange during rest, exercise and sleep in severe chronic obstructive pulmonary disease. *Am Rev Respir Des* 1993;**148**:1030–6.

37 Leitch AG, Hopkin JM, Ellis DA, *et al*. The effect of aerosol ipratropium and salbutamol on exercise in patients with stable fixed chronic bronchitis. *Thorax* 1978;**33**:711–13.

38 Vathinen AS, Britton JR, Ebden P, *et al*. High dose inhaled salbuterol in severe airflow limitation. *Am Rev Respir Dis* 1988;**138**:850–5.

39 Aubier M. Pharmacology of respiratory muscles. *Clin Chest Med* 1988;**9**:311–14.

40 Moxham J. Aminophylline and the respiratory muscles: an alternative view. *Clin Chest Med* 1988;**2**:325–40.

41 Rebuck AS, Chapman KR, Abboud R, *et al*. Nebulised anticholinergic and sympathomimetic treatment of obstructive airways disease in the emergency room. *Am J Med* 1987;**82**:59–64.

42 Combivent Study Group. In chronic obstructive pulmonary disease, a combination of ipratropium and albuterol is more effective that either agent alone. *Chest* 1994;**105**:1411–19.

43 Guyatt GH, Townsend M, Pugsley SO, *et al*. Bronchodilators in chronic airflow limitation effects on airway function, exercise capacity and quality of life. *Am Rev Respir Dis* 1987;**135**:1269–74.

44 Calverley PMA. Symptomatic bronchodilator treatment. In: Calverly PMA, Pride NB (eds), *Chronic obstructive pulmonary disease*. London: Chapman & Hall, 1994:419–46.

45 Jenkins SC, Moxham J. High dose salbutamol in chronic bronchitis comparison of 400 mcg, 1 mg, 1·6 mg, 2 mg and placebo delivered by rotahaler. *Br J Dis Chest* 1987;**81**:242–7.

46 Hansen NCG, Andersen PB. Salbutamol powder inhaled from diskhaler compared to salbutamol inhaled as nebuliser solution in severe chronic airways obstruction. *Respir Med* 1995;**89**:175–80.

47 Sears MR, Rea HH, Beaglehole RG, *et al*. Asthma mortality in New Zealand: a two year national study. *NZ Med J* 1985;**98**:271.

48 van Shayk CP, Dompeling E, van Herwaarden CLA, *et al*. Bronchodilator treatment in moderate asthma or chronic bronchitis: a randomised controlled study. *BMJ* 1991;**303**:1426–31.

49 van Shayk CP, Dompeling E, van Herwaarden CLA, *et al*. Continuous use of bronchodilators versus use on demand in mild asthma and COPD. *Am J Respir Crit Care Med* 1994;**149**:A203.

50 O'Driscoll BR, Taylor RJ, Horsley MG, Chambers DK, Bernstein A. Nebulised salbutamol with and without ipratropium bromide in acute airflow obstruction. *Lancet* 1989;**i**:1418–19.

51 Lim R, Walshaw MJ, Saltissi S, Hind CRK. Cardiac arrhythmias during acute exacerbations of chronic airflow limitation: effect of fall in plasma potassium concentrations induced by nebulised beta agonist therapy. *Postgrad Med J* 1989;**65**:449–52.

52 Smith SR, Ryder CM, Kendall MJ, Holder R. Cardiovascular and biochemical responses to nebulised salbutamol in normal subjects. *Br J Clin Pharmacol* 1984;**18**:641–4.

53 Brashear RE. Arrhythmias in patients with chronic obstructive pulmonary disease. *Med Clin N Am* 1984;**68**:969–81.

54 Jenkins SC, Heaton RW, Fulton TJ, Moxham J. Comparison of domiciliary nebulised salbutamol and salbutamol from a metered dose aerosol in stable COPD. *Chest* 1987;**91**:804–7.

55 Sutton PP, Gemmell RG, Innes N, *et al*. Use of nebulised saline and nebulised terbutaline as an adjunct to chest physiotherapy. *Thorax* 1988;**43**:57–60.

56 *MIMMS* (May) London: Haymarket, 1995.

57 Armitage JM, Williams SJ. Inhaler technique in the elderly. *Age Ageing* 1988;**17**:275–8.

58 Buckley D. Assessment of inhaler technique in general practice. *Irish J Med Sci* 1989:275–99.

59 Diggory P, Bialey R, Vallon A. Effectiveness of inhaled bronchodilator delivery systems for elderly patients. *Age Ageing* 1991;**20**:379–82.

60 Newman SP, Weiz AWB, Talaee N, Clarke SW. Improvement of drug delivery with a breath actuated pressured aerosol for patients with poor inhaler techniques. *Thorax* 1991;**46**:712–16.

61 Ollerenshaw SL, Woolcock AJ. Characteristics of the inflammation in biopsies from large airways of subjects with volume and subjects with chronic airflow limitation. *Ann Rev Respir Dis* 1992;**145**:922–7.

62 Nisar M, Walshaw MJ, Earis JE, Pearson MG, Calverley PMA. Assessment of airway reversibility of airway obstruction in patients with chronic obstructive airways disease. *Thorax* 1990;**45**:190–4.

63 Rimmington LD, Spence DPS, Nisar M, Earis JE, Calverly PMA, Pearson MG. Predictors of 5 year mortality in COPD. *Am Rev Respir Dis* 1993;**147**:A323.

64 Weir DC, Burge PS. Effects of high dose inhaled beclomethasone diprorionate 750 µg and 1500 µg twice daily and 40 mg per day oral prednisolone on lung function, symptoms and bronchial hyperresponsiveness in patients with non-asthmatic chronic airflow obstruction. *Thorax* 1993;**48**:309–16.

65 O'Driscoll BR, Kay EA, Taylor RJ, Bernstein A. Home nebulisers: can optimal therapy be predicted by laboratory studies. *Respir Med* 1990;**84**:170.

66 Hosker H, Cooke NJ, Hawkes P. Antibiotics in chronic obstructive pulmonary disease. *BMJ* 1994;**308**:871–2.

67 Moayyedi P, Congleton J, Page RL, Pearson SB, Muers MH. Comparison of nebulised salbutamol and ipratropium bromide with salbutamol alone in the treatment of chronic obstructive pulmonary disease. *Thorax* 1995;**50**:834–7.

68 Burrows B, Niden AH, Barclay WR, Kasik JE. Chronic obstructive lung disease II. Relationship of the clinical and physiologic findings to the severity of the airways obstruction. *Am Rev Respir Dis* 1965;**92**:665–78.

69 Wynder EL, Kaufman PL, Lesser RL. A short term follow up study of ex-cigarette smokers. *Am Rev Respir Dis* 1967;**96**:665–78.

70 Hirsch SR, Niernes PF, Korg KC. The expectorant effect of glyceryl guiacolate in patients with chronic bronchitis: a controlled in vitro and in vivo study. *Chest* 1973;**63**:9–14.

71 Fazio F, Lafortuna C. Effect of inhaled salbutamol on mucociliary clearance in patients with chronic bronchitis. *Chest* 1981;**80**:827–30.

72 Devalia JL, Sapsford RJ, Rusznak C, *et al.* The effects of salmeterol and salbutamol on ciliary beat frequency of cultured human bronchial epithelial cells in vitro. *Pulmonary Pharmacol* 1992;**5**:257–63.

73 Leifkauf GD, Ueki IF, Nadel JA. Selective autonomic regulation of the viscostatic properties of sub-mucosal gland secretion from cat trachea. *J Appl Physiol* 1984; **56**:26–30.

74 Pearson MG, Ahmad D, Chamberlain MJ, Morgan WKC, Vinitski S. Aminophylline and mucociliary clearance in irreversible airflow limitation. *Br J Clin Pharmacol* 1985;**20**:688–90.

75 Boman G, Backer U, Larsson S, Melander B, Wahlander L. Oral acetyl cysteine reduces exacerbation rates in chronic bronchitis. Report of a trial organised by the Swedish Society of Pulmonary Diseases. *Eur J Respir Dis* 1983;**64**:405–9.

5 Smoking cessation

HEINRICH WORTH

Introduction

Smoking of cigarette tobacco remains the single most important preventable cause of death and of respiratory diseases. Smoking cessation is therefore the key to the prevention and care of patients with chronic obstructive pulmonary disease (COPD). There are two broad management strategies to implement for sustained tobacco abstinence: drug treatments and behavioural intervention. Pharmacological interventions include nicotine replacement, nicotine antagonists, and symptomatic treatment of smoking withdrawal. The Nicotine Polacrilex gum and transdermal nicotine (patch) are the most widely used nicotine substitutes, with the nicotine patch being the first line replacement therapy because it is easier to use and comply with than the gum.

Clonidine, antidepressants, and buspirone require further study to determine what role, if any, they should play in the treatment of nicotine dependence.

Behavioural intervention strategies include the following:

- Self-monitoring
- Goal setting
- Stimulus control or alternative behaviours
- Aversion therapy.

The stages of smoking cessation are precontemplation, contemplation, action, and maintenance; interventions are selected on the basis of the stage at which the smoker is.

84

In general, no one behavioural intervention has been demonstrated as superior in either stimulating cessation or maintaining abstinence. Most successful smoking cessation programmes employ a multicomponent approach with behavioural intervention and nicotine replacement strategies. Combined with the policy of restricting the use of tobacco, primary prevention in youth and adolescents appears to be fundamental to the reduction of morbidity and mortality resulting from smoking.

As a risk factor for lung cancer, chronic obstructive pulmonary disease, cerebrovascular disease, and coronary artery disease, cigarette smoking remains the single most important preventable cause of death and of respiratory diseases. Smoking acts synergistically with a host of occupational and environmental agents to produce lung damage.

Evidence is accumulating to substantiate the harmful effects of involuntary (passive) smoking.[1-3] Passive smoking appears to increase the risk of lung cancer death, heart diseases, and asthma. In children, it worsens the symptoms of asthma, and it increases the risk of middle ear disease.[4]

Finally, the economic health costs of tobacco use are staggering. Average lifetime medical costs for a smoker are estimated to be US$6000 higher than for a non-smoker.[5] Studies have placed the costs of smoking for the United States of America at a US$65 billion in 1985 in terms of health care expenditures and lost productivity.[6]

Pharmacological intervention

Clinical course of nicotine addiction

One third to one half of occasional cigarette smokers graduate to maladaptive use and to physical dependence on nicotine.[11] At this point, the disorder is chronic. The effects of nicotine that are associated with dependence include increased expression of brain nicotine receptors, changes in regional brain glucose metabolism, electroencephalographic changes, the release of catecholamines, tolerance, and physiological dependence.[12] These effects increase the compulsion to smoke by producing positive reinforcement (with the administration of nicotine) and withdrawal symptoms (with abstinence).[12]

85

Withdrawal symptoms (restlessness, irritability, anxiety, drowsiness, sleep disturbances, impatience, confusion, impaired concentration, and weight loss) are intensified by abrupt abstinence from nicotine beginning within a few hours, peaking within a few hours, and typically lasting for four weeks, although there is considerable variability.[13]

Pharmacokinetic considerations

Cigarette smoke must be inhaled to be absorbed effectively in the pulmonary alveoli, where absorption of nicotine is rapid.[11] From the lung, nicotine is absorbed into alveolar capillary blood and carried to the heart, and then to the brain and other organs. Thus, peak arterial plasma nicotine concentrations may be 10 times greater than venous concentrations (see Henningfield[14]).

Cigarettes contain 6–11 mg nicotine, of which the smoker typically absorbs 1–3 mg (see Henningfield[14]). The typical pack per day smoker absorbs 20–40 mg nicotine each day, achieving plasma concentrations of 25–35 mg/ml by the afternoon.[11] The plasma half life of nicotine is about 2 hours.[15]

Benefits of stopping smoking

The health benefits of smoking cessation are substantial. With few exceptions, risks of disease decline with smoking cessation and continue to drop as the period of abstinence lengthens.[7] After 10–15 years of abstinence, the overall risk of mortality approximates that of people who have never smoked.[8] The risk of coronary heart disease and the risk of stroke diminish soon after a smoker quits and largely disappears in 2–4 years (see Haxby[9]). Virtually all types of smoking related cancers occur less frequently in ex-smokers with long term abstinence than in smokers. After 10 years of abstinence the risk of lung cancer is reduced by 50–70%.[8]

Smoking cessation is associated with rapid reduction in coughing, phlegm production, and wheezing, and former smokers have a lower death rate from influenza and pneumonia.[8] Smoking cessation slows the decline in pulmonary function to the same rates as in non-smokers, and if smokers quit before they have developed COPD, they are less likely to develop the disease than those who continue to smoke.[8] Many smokers are not aware of the dramatic benefits of quitting. It is critical that they are educated about these. Emphasising the substantial benefits of quitting may help motivation.

Smoking cessation programmes

Most smoking cessation programmes are generally quite effective in helping people to stop smoking, but only temporarily. Although smoking cessation rates at post-treatment typically range from 70% to 90%, up to 80% of those smokers who initially succeed in stopping smoking eventually relapse over the 12 month period following initial cessation (see Carmody[10]). Therefore, the greater challenge in smoking cessation is maintenance of abstinence beyond the phase of acute withdrawal and for extended periods thereafter.

It should be emphasised that people do not stop smoking for intellectual reasons; they stop smoking for personal and emotional reasons such as advanced loss of lung function, which means loss of health, recreational pursuits, job, and sexual function.

There are two broad management strategies that need to be implemented for sustained tobacco abstinence: drug treatments including nicotine replacement and behavioural intervention.

Pharmacological interventions

Three pharmacological approaches have received significant attention: nicotine replacement, nicotine antagonists (blockade therapy), and symptomatic treatment of smoking withdrawal.

Nicotine replacement

Nicotine medications make it easier to abstain from tobacco by replacing, at least partially, the nicotine formerly obtained from tobacco. As the medications described in this paper are not capable of producing the high arterial or even the lower venous plasma concentrations typical of tobacco use, the description of the treatment as "replacement medication" is misleading.

Nicotine medications reduce withdrawal symptoms which occur in about 80% of smokers during smoking cessation. They partially satiate the appetite for cigarettes by sustaining tolerance (see Henningfield[14]). Finally, they may provide some of the effects for which the patient previously relied on cigarettes, such as sustaining desirable mood and attentional states, and making it easier to handle stressful situations.

Nicotine medications—The first nicotine medication used was a transmucosally delivered product, Nicotine Polacrilex ("nicotine gum"). It is available in a dose of 2 or 4 mg nicotine per piece. Ten to twelve doses per day provide about 10 mg/day from the 2 mg form and 20 mg/day from the 4 mg form, or about one third to one half the usual daily intake of a person who smokes 30 cigarettes a day.[16] Ninety per cent of the biologically available nicotine in the gum can be released over 20–40 min. Absorption is reduced when acidic beverages such as coffee or soft drinks are consumed while Nicotine Polacrilex is being used.[17] If it is chewed too rapidly, local or systemic toxicity will occur. Local effects are irritation or anaesthesia of the buccal or pharyngeal mucosa, jaw ache, and a sore throat. Acute systemic toxicity is manifested by lightheadedness, nausea, salivation, vomiting and diarrhoea. Contraindications to its use include pregnancy, lactation, known cardiac arrhythmia or recent myocardial infarction, severe angina, peptic ulcer, and any significant temporomandibular joint disease.

The transdermal route of nicotine medication may theoretically have three significant advantages over chewing gum:

1 It avoids the bad taste and gastrointestinal symptoms associated with the chewing gum
2 The transdermal approach provides continuous nicotine delivery that is less reliant on patient compliance
3 It can be used in some patients for whom the gum is contraindicated (peptic ulcers, dentures). However, transdermal nicotine patches which usually contain 11–22 mg nicotine, deliver about 0·9 mg nicotine/hour; achieving maximal systemic doses requires 2–3 days, at which time plasma nicotine concentrations are generally lower than in a pack per day smoker.[19]

Thus the transition from smoking to medication may be associated with a rapid reduction in plasma nicotine concentrations in heavy smokers.

Two additional systems are undergoing clinical testing: one, a nasal spray that delivers 0·5 mg nicotine per pulse, can be used repeatedly to deliver higher doses quickly.[20] The other is an oral inhaler that provides 0·01 mg nicotine to the buccal mucosa and throat when a 35 ml puff is inhaled through a mouthpiece. It cannot easily be used to achieve the systematic doses produced by tobacco or the other nicotine preparations.[21]

Efficacy—Nicotine Polacrilex and transdermal medications are efficacious in helping smokers abstain from tobacco,[22-25] including clinics run by psychologists,[26 27] general medical practices,[28] inpatient programmes,[29] and hospital based clinics which treat patients with smoking related diseases.[23] An important determinant of efficacy appears to be the ancillary support provided to patients: in studies in which the nicotine gum was simply dispensed,[30] or was provided without extensive guidance,[31] the rates of cessation of smoking were those of untreated patients.

The rates of cessation during the first few months of treatment with transdermal preparations typically range from 20% to 40%.[25] These rates are about twice those achieved by patients given placebo and three times those of patients who try to quit smoking without any form of therapy.

The long and short term rates are generally lower in general medical practices than in smoking cessation clinics. In one study, in a general practice setting, the rates of abstinence in the nicotine and placebo groups at two years were 12% and 3%, respectively.[32]

Although it may appear that transdermal nicotine is more effective than Nicotine Polacrilex, no trial has compared the two medications directly. Many of the trials of nicotine gum were conducted during the early and mid 1980s when there was less social support for abstinence from tobacco and less efficient behavioural intervention strategies than when studies of transdermal nicotine were conducted. For both nicotine medications it should be emphasised that treated patients remain susceptible to relapse.

Promising data have also been obtained in placebo controlled studies of nicotine nasal spray and oral vapour inhalers.[20 21] These formulations may extend the range of patients who can be effectively treated with nicotine medications.

Recommendations on dosing—The essential elements of therapy with nicotine medications are diagnosis, rational dosing, appropriate warnings, and follow up. There is a general correlation between the level of dependence, scores on the Fagerström test (an index of nicotine dependence) (Table 5.1) or markers of nicotine intake, and the probable severity of withdrawal symptoms, degree of difficulty in achieving abstinence, and speed of relapse (see Henningfield[14]).

As a starting point for dosing, patients should be given one dose of 2 mg Nicotine Polacrilex in place of every two cigarettes. For patients who smoke more than 20 cigarettes per day or whose

Table 5.1   The Fagerström Test for Nicotine Dependence[33]

Questions and answers	Score
How soon after you wake up do you smoke Your first cigarette?	
≤ 5 min	3
6–30 min	2
31–60 min	1
≥ 61 min	0
Do you find it difficult to refrain from smoking in places where it is forbidden—for example, in church, at the library, in a cinema?	
Yes	1
No	0
Which cigarette would you hate most to give up?	
The first in the morning	1
Any other	0
How many cigarettes per day do you smoke?	
≤ 10	0
11–20	1
21–30	2
≥ 31	3
Do you smoke more frequently during the first hours after waking than during the rest of the day?	
Yes	1
No	0
Do you smoke if you are so ill that you are in bed most of the day?	
Yes	1
No	0

Scores of more than 6 are generally interpreted as indicating a high degree of dependence, with more severe withdrawal symptoms, greater difficulty in quitting, and possibly the need for higher doses of medication.

Fagerström scores are above 6,[33] one dose of 4 mg Nicotine Polacrilex should be described in place of every three to four cigarettes. Patients with inadequate relief of withdrawal symptoms should be encouraged to increase the number of doses per day. After one or two months, weaning can be initiated, with the total daily intake decreased by one unit dose each week.

For transdermal nicotine, people who smoke more than 10 cigarettes per day should be treated with the highest available dose of the brand used. After one or two months of treatment at the initial dose, weaning can begin, with each of the lower dosages prescribed for 2–4 weeks. Patients who smoke fewer than 10 cigarettes per day should begin with a mid-range transdermal dose.

People who smoke five or fewer cigarettes per day appear to have a low level of dependence. They may or may not benefit from nicotine replacement therapy.

Instructions for proper use—If Nicotine Polacrilex is prescribed, patients should practise the proper techniques for use before they quit smoking. They need to learn to compress the gum a few times with their teeth, then let it rest in the mouth, repeating every minute or so for 15–20 min per dose. The prescription should specify a fixed dosing schedule and should include instructions not to use the medication while consuming beverages (see Henningfield[14]).

If the transdermal route is prescribed, application sites should be discussed to ensure the choice of a hairless site that will be comfortable with clothing. Changing the site each day will reduce the risk of skin irritation which occurs in 35–45% of patch users. Other less common adverse effects associated with the nicotine patch are sleep disturbance, gastrointestinal complaints, dizziness, and sweating.

Combination therapy with nicotine gum and transdermal nicotine—The combination of transdermal nicotine and Nicotine Polacrilex may have enhanced efficacy in relieving withdrawal symptoms and achieving cessation.[34 35] The rationale for combined therapy is that the transdermal system ensures a stable intake of nicotine which can be supplemented with Nicotine Polacrilex in response to momentary need. The long term benefits of combined therapy are not known, but such therapy appears to be reasonable in patients who have not responded to other types of treatment and those who are highly dependent on nicotine.

Nicotine antagonists

Drugs blocking the effects of nicotine could theoretically be used as anti-smoking aids. Although unlikely to aid initial cessation, they may have a role in preventing relapse, by suppressing the reinforcement obtained by smoking. For mecylamine and β blockers,[36] no convincing positive effects on smoking cessation have been observed.

Symptomatic treatment of nicotine withdrawal

Clonidine appears to have an effective role in the management of nicotine withdrawal.[37] It reduces withdrawal symptoms including alleviation of craving, anxiety, irritability, restlessness, and tension. The mechanism by which clonidine achieves its therapeutic effect is not known. Oral clonidine hydrochloride can be given at 0·05 mg/

day initially, and the dosage can be adjusted up to 0·3 mg/day, administered in divided doses. Alternatively, the clonidine transdermal system (patch) can be used at a dosage of 0·1–0·2 mg/day. As clonidine frequently has adverse effects[38 39] and has questionable effectiveness, its role in smoking cessation should be limited. However, it is reasonable to try this agent in combination with nicotine substitution and behavioural therapy in individuals who fail to respond to nicotine replacement.

Other drugs

Another widely used drug in smoking cessation is lobeline, commercially marketed in "over the counter" preparations. Controlled studies indicate that lobeline preparations are no more effective in short term cessation efforts than placebos and have no long term abstinence benefit.

Substantial evidence is accumulating that cigarette smokers have a higher prevalence of depression and anxiety than non-smokers.[40] These findings have stimulated interest in anxiolytics and antidepressants as possible treatments for nicotine dependence.[41] To date, only preliminary studies on the role of these drugs in smoking cessation have been published.

Although the results of studies on benzodiazepines are not encouraging,[42] buspirone seems more promising.[43] Studies on buspirone in subjects who have relapsed as a result of negative mood during previous attempts at quitting are, however, needed. Until more is known, buspirone should be reserved for smokers with other problems, for example, anxiety.

Hypnosis and acupuncture

In controlled studies, very high success rates (45–85%) have been claimed for hypnotherapy or acupuncture. Well designed clinical trials with success rates of only 20% or less do not support these claims. The reported success rates in controlled studies on hypnosis therapy are not higher than the expected proportion of the population susceptible to hypnosis, or than that reported for alternative smoking cessation modalities.

The best available data[44] imply that acupuncture offers no significant advantage concerning short term and long term abstinence rates compared with behavioural intervention strategies including nicotine replacement.

Behavioural intervention strategies

The most effective formal behavioural approaches employ cessation management and relapse prevention programmes targeted at the act of smoking itself or at conditions and circumstances that elicit, prompt, or determine smoking initiation (such as anxiety, stress, and social and personal environment). The components of behavioural intervention include: (1) self monitoring; (2) goal setting or contracting; (3) stimulus control or alternative behaviours; and (4) aversion.

Self monitoring

The observation of one's own behaviour can provide a useful baseline against which to measure change. It also increases awareness of smoking behaviour and provides information about smoking patterns. The method should not be overly complex, the targets of monitoring should vary, and the monitoring should not always focus on negative "targets" such as the experience of withdrawal symptoms, but should include the positive benefits of non-smoking such as a reduced loss of lung function.

Goal setting or contracting

Setting a specific target date for quitting in the near future is a frequent programme component. All smoking cessation programmes involve implicit or explicit contracts by the participants to quit smoking or reduce consumption. These contracts only last as long as they are in effect, however, and relapse tends to occur after the contract period has passed. Thus, unless the participant is willing to enter very long term contracts, additional relapse prevention components are needed.

Stimulus control or alternative behaviours

To break the environmental association of smoking, stimulus control is used for progressive narrowing of the range of situations when smoking might occur and to reduce consumption. Developing alternative behaviours is a method of coping with the urge of smoking. Participants should be encouraged to develop a range of behaviours so that back up strategies are available if the first

93

alternative fails or if it is impossible to perform under the circumstances. Exercise, for example, is a desirable substitute for its cardiovascular benefits and mood enhancement.

Aversion therapies

Aversion therapies aim to reduce the pleasurable effects of smoking and are designed to capitalise on the naturally occurring immediate negative features. Three types of aversive stimuli have been employed. Electric shock has not been shown to be effective in promoting cessation. In overt sensitisation the smoker is asked to imagine one or more unpleasant scenes or scripts when smoking or when experiencing the urge to smoke. The expectation is that smoking will prompt unpleasant thought and associated feelings, and that such states will block the act, if not the urge, to smoke on subsequent occasions. In overt sensitisation or directed smoking procedure, smokers are instructed to use a smoking protocol that will intensify unpleasant features. Rapid cigarette smoking is an aversive procedure and one of the most effective techniques yet identified for producing abstinence.[45] Subjects are instructed to take a puff of the cigarette every 6 seconds until they cannot tolerate any more. Subjects often become nauseated by the procedure, although not usually to the point of vomiting. The procedure may be used from one to 12 sessions. Trials that have used rapid smoking have reported rates of cessation of 50–60% at six months or a year.[45 46]

Concerns have been about the safety of rapid smoking, primarily based on the possibility of nicotine poisoning and cardiovascular stress. Sachs et al[47] have reviewed the literature on rapid smoking and have compared the risks and benefits of rapid smoking wth the risks and effects for healthy subjects. For patients with mild to moderate cardiac and pulmonary disease, however, rapid smoking might be dangerous.

A variant of the nicotine toxicity aversion induced by oversmoking is to deliver warm stale smoke into the face of the smoker who is rapidly smoking. Controlled studies in this technique are limited, but promising, with 40–60% abstinence rates at the end of one year.

In general, aversion techniques by themselves do not induce long term abstinence. Unfortunately, the most effective protocols can produce damaging physical (and perhaps, psychological) side effects and, as such, place important limitations on the efficacy of aversion techniques.

Determinants of outcome

Over the years, many programmes have appeared with an initial success rate of about 70–80% cessation of smoking rate, but end with over 80% or greater long term failure rate.[48 49] Demography, personal factors, social factors, and biological factors are determinants of outcome in smoking cessation.[50] The analysis of Lennox[50] revealed the following main results:

1 Women generally find it more difficult to give up smoking than men. With respect to men, women were more dependent on cigarettes, were more likely to cut down consumption than to stop completely, and were less confident in being able to stop smoking.

2 Most studies which have examined socioeconomic factors have found no association with outcome.

3 The evidence of many studies is conclusive that heavier smokers find it more difficult to stop. There might be a major addictive component to heavy smoking which makes giving up more difficult. Besides Fagerström's eight point tolerance questionnaire (see Table 5.1), a valid measure of addiction can be simply obtained from the number of cigarettes smoked per day and the time from waking to the first cigarette of the day.[51]

4 A greater belief in personal control of one's life, as opposed to control by fate, was associated with a better outcome.

5 Stopping for financial reasons predicted a poor outcome, whereas stopping because of a desire to improve one's health predicted a good outcome.[52 53]

6 The evidence suggests that those who smoke for reasons of addiction and habit are less likely to stop smoking.[53]

7 Stress has been shown to be adversely associated with both short term and long term cessation, respectively.[54]

8 Recent research into cessation has focused on the role of coping skills, both cognitive and behavioural, in preventing relapse. The use of multiple coping skills was found to be associated with long term abstinence.

9 Several studies have shown that the support of others (for example, partners) enhances outcome. Almost all analyses of relapse situations have found an adverse relationship between outcome and the number of smokers in the environment.

10 Alcohol consumption and a specific crisis (for example, family crisis, work related crisis) in the ex-smoker's social situation are reasons for relapse.

Table 5.2 Effects of selected patient characteristics on attempts at stopping smoking and possible interventions

Characteristics	Association with better outcome	Interventions
Addiction		
Daily cigarette consumption	Lower consumption	Encourage to cut down "non-essential" cigarettes before date for stopping completely; a smoking diary may be useful
Cigarette withdrawal symptoms	Fewer symptoms	Consider use of nicotine medication particularly for heavier smokers
Personal factors		
Self efficacy, expectation of success, confidence	Higher levels	Give encouragement; promote self esteem; build on any previous success
Appreciation of health risks	Better appreciation	Emphasise health consequences of stopping/continuing smoking; consider use of oximeter or flowmeter
Desire to stop smoking	More desire	Reinforce benefits of stopping and risks of not stopping
Motives for stopping smoking	Health motive; finance not sole motive	Find out reasons for stopping and reinforce with additional ones, particularly if finance is the only motive offered
Stress	Less stress	Examination of lifestyle; counselling; relaxation techniques
Coping skills	Better skills	Anticipate relapse situations and plan behavioural or cognitive responses in advance; leaflets may be useful
Social factors		
Social support	More support	Encourage to involve others: asking partner to stop, telling friends and workmates and asking for their support
Smoking status of contacts	Fewer smokers	Encourage to avoid company of other smokers as far as possible
Relapse situations	Less contact with "high risk" situations	Advise to anticipate and avoid high risk situations where possible, and teach use of coping skills
Biological factors		
Weight gain	Less concern over weight gain	Advise choice of oral substitutes, temporary nature of weight gain, benefits of exercise, balance of health risks of smoking and weight gain

Adapted in a modified form from Lennox.[50]

11 Biological factors such as withdrawal symptoms, weight gain have been shown to predict poorer outcome in cessation programmes.

Maintenance strategies

The relapse during smoking cessation periods frequently occurs in situations in which there is social pressure to smoke or in times of frustration.[55] By incorporating interventions with respect to selected patient characteristics (see Table 5.1), as well as training of relapse prevention skills into multicomponent smoking cessation programmes, promising results can be obtained.[18 56 57] In general, no one behaviour intervention has been demonstrated as superior in either stimulating cessation or maintaining abstinence. The success of the different smoking cessation strategies cannot be precisely predicted. Most successful smoking cessation programmes employ a multicomponent treatment approach with behavioural interventions and nicotine replacement strategies.

Individual versus group counselling

To help patients stop smoking physicians should provide a model of healthy lifestyle. Physicians who smoke counsel patients significantly less than physicians who do not smoke.[58 59] For primary care intervention Schwartz[49] calculated a median success rate of 6% after one year for 12 different interventions which consisted of advice only, compared with 23% for 10 studies where interventions consisted of advice plus other components. The higher success rate of 36% for smoking cessation clinics may result from the fact that clinic attenders are a self selected population, motivated to stop smoking. It may also reflect the greater experience and expertise of clinic staff using generally more intensive interventions.

Group counselling is more cost effective than individual counselling and has comparable long term success rates. Group approaches to smoking cessation enhance the development of insight of the participants through peer interchange and enable peer support.

Markers of smoking cessation

Nicotine and carbon monoxide (CO) are the most frequently used biological markers for assessing the delivery of main-stream or side-stream smoke to humans. Of these nicotine is unique to tobacco. Most analyses for quantifying nicotine, or its important stable breakdown product cotinine, in serum or urine are performed by radioimmunoassay (RIA) or gas chromatography. RIA is simple to use, relatively inexpensive, and usually requires small sample volumes. With respect to gas chromatography its shortcoming is lack of specificity, resulting primarily from cross reaction between nicotine and cotinine or other endogenous products common to human fluids.

As CO is generated from the burning of a vast array of organic materials as well as being generated endogenously in humans, it is not unique to tobacco smoke. Therefore, it is a very poor specific biological marker for passive exposure to environmental tobacco smoke. As it is bound too tightly to haemoglobin and released so slowly in exhaled breath, it is also a poor biological marker for assessing the intensity of smoking or for quantifying smoke dosimetry.

Perspective

Most public policies implemented by anti-smoking movements are designed to discourage smoking and tobacco use directly. They promote an anti-smoking message either through education about the potential health hazards of smoking or by creating economic disadvantages to smoking. In more recent years, the policy of restricting the use of tobacco, especially by restriction of smoking in public places, has had a greater impact on reducing tobacco use than all other modalities combined.

Primary prevention efforts have focused principally on the young. The evaluation of such programmes revealed that attitudes and knowledge about drugs and tobacco were effectively altered, but use patterns were not significantly changed. The search for wide reaching and economically feasible programmes that can reduce demand among risk groups should be a continuing priority for those committed to the view that prevention of use is a fundamental key to reduction of morbidity and mortality related to smoking. The most promising approaches include personal and social skill training based on cognitive–behavioural theories of development and stress management.

1 Mahajan VK, Huber GL. Health effects of involuntary smoking: impact on tobacco use, smoking cessation, and public policies. *Semin Respir Med* 1990; **11**:87–114.

2 Weiss ST, Tager IB, Schenker M, Speizer F. The health effect of involuntary smoking. *Am Rev Respir Dis* 1983;**128**:933–42.

3 Celermajer DS, Adams MR, Clarkson P, *et al*. Passive smoking and impaired endothelium dependent arterial dilatation in healthy young adults. *N Engl J Med* 1996;**334**:150–4.

4 Office of Health and Environmental Assessment. *Respiratory health effects of passive smoking: lung cancer, and other disorders.* Washington DC: US Environmental Protection Agency, 1992.

5 Satcher D, Eriksen M. The paradox of tobacco control. *JAMA* 1994;**271**:627–8.

6 MacKenzie TD, Bartecchi E, Schrier RW. The human costs of tobacco use (second of two parts). *N Engl J Med* 1994;**330**:975–80.

7 Samet JM. The health benefits of smoking cessation. *Med Clin North Am* 1992; **76**:399–414.

8 US Department of Health and Human Services. *The health benefits of smoking cessation: a report of the Surgeon General.* Rockville, MD: US Department of Health and Human Services. DHHS publication no. (CDC) 90-8416, 1990.

9 Haxby DN. Treatment of nicotine dependence. *Am J Health-Syst Pharm* 1995; **52**:265–81.

10 Carmody TP. Preventing relapse in the treatment of nicotine addition: current issues and future directions. *J Psychoact Drugs* 1992;**24**:131–58.

11 Department of Health and Human Services. *The health consequences of smoking: nicotine addiction: a report of the Surgeon General.* Washington DC: Government Printing Office DHHS publication no (CDC) 88-8406, 1988.

12 Henningfield JE, Schuh LM, Jarvik ME. Pathophysiology of tobacco dependence. In: Bloom FE, Kupfer DJ, eds. *Psychopharmacology: the fourth generation of progress.* New York: Raven Press, 1990.

13 Hughes JR, Higgins ST, Hatsukami D. Effects of abstinence from tobacco. In: Kozlowski LT, Annis HM, Cappel HD, *et al*, eds. *Research advances in alcohol and drug problems.* New York: Plenum Press, 1990:317–98.

14 Henningfield JE. Nicotine medications for smoking cessation. *N Engl J Med* 1995;**333**:1196–203.

15 Benowitz NL, Jacob P, Denaro C, Jenkins R. Stable isotope studies of nicotine kinetics and bioavailability. *Clin Pharmacol Ther* 1991;**49**:270–7.

16 Benowitz NL. Nicotine replacement therapy: what has been accomplished—can we do better? *Drugs* 1993;**45**:157–70.

17 Henningfield JE, Radzius A, Cooper TM, Clayton RR. Drinking coffee and carbonated beverages, blocks absorption of nicotine from nicotine polacrilex gum. *JAMA* 199;**264**:1560–4.

18 Benowitz NL. Pharmacologic aspects of cigarette smoking and nicotine addition. *N Engl J Med* 1988;**319**:1318–30.

19 Ross HD, Chan KK, Piraino AJ, John VA. Pharmacokinetics of multiple daily transdermal doses of nicotine in healthy smokers. *Pharmacol Res* 1991;**8**:385–8.

20 Sutherland G, Stapleton JA, Russel MAH, *et al*. Randomized controlled trial of nasal nicotine spray in smoking cessation. *Lancet* 1992;**340**:324–9.

21 Toennessen P, Noerregaard J, Mikkelsen K, Joergensen S, Nilsson F. A double blind trial of a nicotine inhaler for smoking cessation. *JAMA* 1993;**269**:1268–71.

22 Malcolm RE, Sillett RW, Turner JA, Ball KP. The use of nicotine chewing gum as an aid to stop smoking. *Psychopharmacology* 1980;**70**:295–6.

23 Hjalmarson AIM. Effect of nicotine chewing gum in smoking cessation; a randomized, placebo-controlled, double-blind study. *JAMA* 1984;**252**:2835–8.

24 Silagy C, Mant D, Fowler G, Lokge M. Meta-analysis on efficacy of nicotine replacement therapies in smoking cessation. *Lancet* 1994;**343**:139–42.

25 Fiore MC, Smith SS, Jorenby DE, Baker TB. The effectiveness of the nicotine patch for smoking cessation: a meta-analysis. *JAMA* 1994;**271**:1940–7.
26 Hall SM, Tunstall C, Rugg D, Jones RT, Benowitz NL. Nicotine gum and behavioral treatment in smoking cessation. *J Consult Clin Psychol* 1985;**53**: 256–8.
27 Harvis MJ, Raw M, Russel MAH, Feyerabend C. Randomised controlled trial of nicotine chewing gum. *BMJ* 1982;**285**:537–40.
28 Sachs DPL, Säwe U, Leischow SJ. Effectiveness of a 16-hour transdermal nicotine patch in a medical practise setting, without intensive group counseling. *Arch Intern Med* 1993;**53**:1881–90.
29 Hurt RD, Dale LC, Offort KP, Bruce BK, McCain FL, Eberman KM. Inpatient treatment of severe nicotine dependence. *Mayo Clin Proc* 1992;**67**:823–8.
30 Schneider NG, Jarvik ME, Forsythe AB, Read LL, Elliott ML, Schweiger A. Nicotine gum in smoking cessation: a placebo controlled, double blind trial. *Addict Behav* 1983;**8**:253–61.
31 The Research Committee of the British Thoracic Society. Comparison of four methods of smoking withdrawal in patients with smoking related diseases. *BMJ* 1983;**286**:595–7.
32 Toennessen P, Noerregaard J, Säwe U. Two-year outcome in a smoking cessation trial with a nicotine patch. *J Smok Relat Disord* 1992;**3**:241–5.
33 Heatherton TF, Kozlowzki LT, Frecker RC, Fagerström KO. The Fagerström test for nicotine dependence: a revision of the Fagerström Tolerance Questionnaire. *Br J Addict* 1991;**86**:1119–27.
34 Fagerström KO, Schneider NE, Lunell E. Effectiveness of nicotine patch and nicotine gum as individual versus combined treatments for tobacco withdrawal symptoms. *Psychopharmacology* 1993;**111**:271–7.
35 Kornitzer KM, Boutsen M, Dramaix M, Thijs J, Gustavsson G. Combined use of nicotine patch and gum in smoking cessation: a placebo-controlled clinical trial. *Prev Med* 1995;**24**:41–7.
36 Dow RJ, Fee WM. Use of beta-blocking agents with group therapy in a smoking withdrawal clinic. *J R Soc Med* 1984;**77**:648.
37 Glassman AH, Stetner F, Walsh T, *et al.* Heavy smokers, smoking cessation and clonidine. *JAMA* 1988;**259**:2863–6.
38 Gourlay S, Forbes A, Marriner T, *et al.* A placebo-controlled study of three clonidine doses for smoking cessation. *Clin Pharmacol Ther* 1994;**55**:64–9.
39 Prochazka AV, Petty TL, Nett L, *et al.* Transdermal clonidine reduced withdrawal symptoms but did not increase smoking cessation. *Arch Intern Med* 1992;**152**: 2065–9.
40 Breslau N, Kilbey MM, Andreski P. Vulnerability to psychopathology in nicotine dependent smokers: an epidemiologic study of young adults. *Am J Psychiatry* 1993;**150**:941–9.
41 Hall SM, Munoz RF, Reus VI, *et al.* Nicotine, negative effect and depression. *J Consult Clin Psychol* 1993;**61**:761–7.
42 Robbins AS. Pharmacological approaches to smoking cessation. *Am J Prev Med* 1993;**9**:31–3.
43 Hillemann DD, Mohiuddin SM, Del Core MG, *et al.* Effect of buspirone on withdrawal symptoms associated with smoking cessation. *Arch Intern Med* 1992; **152**:350–2.
44 Aiping J, Meng C. Analysis of therapeutic effects of acupuncture on abstinence from smoking. *J Trad Clin Med* 1994;**14**:56–63.
45 Lichtenstein E, Harris DE, Birchler GR, Wahl JM, Schmuhl DP. Comparison of rapid smoking, warm smokey air and attention placebo in the modification of smoking behaviour. *J Consult Clin Psychol* 1973;**40**:92–8.
46 Best JA, Bass F, Owen LE. Mode of service delivery in a smoking cessation program for public health. *Can J Public Health* 1977;**68**:469–73.

47 Sachs DPL, Pechazek TF, Hall RG, Fitzgerald J. Clarification of risk–benefit issues in rapid smoking. *J Consult Clin Psychol* 1979;**47**:1053–60.
48 Health and Public Policy Committee, American College of Physicians. Methods for stopping smoking. *Ann Intern Med* 1986;**105**:281–91.
49 Schwartz JL. *Review and evaluation of smoking cessation methods: The United States and Canada, 1978–1985.* NIH, Pub No 87:2940,1980.
50 Lennox AS. Determinants of outcome in smoking cessation. *Br J Gen Pract* 1992;**42**:247–52.
51 Heatherton TF, Kozlowzki LT, Frecker RC, *et al.* Measuring the heaviness of smoking; using self-reported time to the first cigarette of the day and number of cigarettes smoked per day. *Br J Addict* 1989;**84**:791–9.
52 Eisinger RA. Psychosocial predictors of smoking recidivism. *J Health Soc Behav* 1971;**12**:355–62.
53 Eisinger RA. Psychosocial predictors of smoking behaviour change. *Soc Sci Med* 1972;**6**:137–44.
54 Ockene JK, Benfari RC, Nutall RL, *et al.* Relationship of psychosocial factors to smoking behaviour change in an intervention program. *Prev Med* 1982;**11**: 13–28.
55 Shiffman S. Relapse following smoking cessation: a situational analysis. *J Consult Clin Psychol* 1982;**50**:71–86.
56 Hall SM, Rugg P, Tunstall C, Jones RT. Preventing relapse to cigarette smoking by behavioural skill training. *J Consult Clin Psychol* 1984;**55**:372–82.
57 Killen JD, Maccoby N, Taylor CB. Nicotine gum and self regulation training in smoking relapse prevention. *Behav Ther* 1984;**15**:234–48.
58 Anda RF, Remington PL, Sienko DG, Davis RM. Are physicians advising smokers to quit? *JAMA* 1987;**257**:1916–19.
59 Folsom AR, Grimm RH. Stop smoking advice by physicians: a feasible approach? *Am J Public Health* 1987;**77**:849–50.

6 Physiotherapy for the patient with COPD

JENNIFER A PRYOR, BARBARA A WEBBER

An individually tailored comprehensive rehabilitation programme can make the difference between a fulfilling life and a life of pulmonary disability.

Rodrigues and Ilowite (1993)[1]

A pulmonary rehabilitation programme aims to reverse the disability resulting from lung disease rather than attempting to reverse the chronic progressive disease process,[2] and should improve quality of life. In patients with chronic obstructive pulmonary disease (COPD) breathlessness is the most disabling symptom, leading to decreasing activity. As the level of fitness deteriorates, a vicious circle of breathlessness and ever decreasing activity is set up. The fear of breathlessness, the inability to carry out normal daily tasks, and the reduced quality of life lead to anxiety and depression. Characteristics of patients who have benefited from pulmonary rehabilitation programmes include those who recognise that they have some disability or impairment associated with their lung disease and are well motivated because of their desire to improve their health status.[2][3]

As has been indicated in previous chapters, the goals for each patient must be realistic. Identification of the general and physiotherapeutic goals for an individual should be in collaboration with members of the pulmonary rehabilitation team to ensure that the benefits that the patient hopes to achieve and the expectations of the patient's family/carer and the rehabilitation team are the same.[4] Unachievable goals demotivate not only the individual, but also the group as a whole.

Assessment

Medical assessment

Before entering a pulmonary rehabilitation programme medical assessment is recommended (see chapter 10). This will identify the severity of patients' symptoms and the effects that their condition have on their lifestyle. It also provides an opportunity to assess the patient's drug therapy and to ensure that this is optimal before starting the programme. Investigations may include pulmonary function testing, measurement of arterial blood gases, electrocardiogram and exercise tests, chest radiograph, and sputum culture. These tests contribute objective information but may not be measures of disability, for example, forced expiratory volume in one second (FEV_1) is not a predictor of disability.[5]

Endurance tests, for example, maximal oxygen uptake, treadmill walking, or the shuttle walking test,[6] can be used to determine maximal endurance. A percentage of this is taken in setting the level for exercise, which may be set at 50%,[7] although it could be higher when a "gold" standard endurance test is established for patients with COPD. The shuttle walking test has been shown to correlate with maximal oxygen uptake.[8]

Physiotherapy assessment

It is essential for the physiotherapist to identify the individual patient's problems. A concise summary should be obtained from the patient's medical notes, including results of pulmonary function tests, sputum culture, blood gases, and chest radiographs.

Subjective information from the patient should include recent history, current problems, presence of cough, sputum, breathlessness, wheeze or chest pain, smoking status, support at home, physical difficulties at home such as climbing stairs, occupation, and hobbies.

Objective data should be obtained on age, sex, height, weight, colour and quantity of sputum, pattern of breathing, chest wall shape and movement, breath sounds on auscultation, arterial oxygen saturation at rest and on exercise, exercise ability, and quality of life.

Exercise testing

Walking tests have evolved as simple measures of exercise ability. They are easy to undertake and require inexpensive equipment.

The 12 minute walking test[9] and six minute walking test[10] are self paced walking tests which require the subject to walk up and down a corridor of known length for a period of either 12 or six minutes. By the end of the test the subject should feel unable to have covered any further distance.

The shuttle walking test is externally paced and therefore less dependent on the patient's motivation and encouragement from the observer.[6] The test is incremental and progressive with the individual being stressed to a maximal performance limited by symptoms. The subject walks a 10 metre course around two marker cones, the speed being dictated by instructions and audiosignals from a cassette tape recording;[6] the test is reproducible after one practice walk. This test has been shown to correlate with maximal oxygen uptake[8] and with the "Breathing Problems Questionnaire" (BPQ).[11] The "Chronic Respiratory Disease Questionnaire" (CRDQ)[12] does not correlate with the shuttle test and this may be a reflection of the greater emphasis of the CRDQ on psychological problems.

Exercise tests should be used in conjunction with measures of perceived exertion and breathlessness. Using the modified Borg scale at the end of the test[13 14] the patient can be asked to rate the maximum level of perceived respiratory effort during the test. A visual analogue scale can be used as an objective measure of the individual's breathlessness before and after the exercise test to establish a frame of reference for the test. The subjective feeling of breathlessness within the same patient may vary.

Quality of life measures

Health Related Quality of Life (HRQL) questionnaires can be used as assessment tools for a patient entering a pulmonary rehabilitation programme.[15] Disease specific questionnaires include the BPQ, the CRDQ, and the St George's Respiratory Questionnaire (SGRQ).[16] These can be used on their own or may be combined with a general health questionnaire to assess the effects in a broader context. The advantages and disadvantages of these measures are discussed in chapter 9.

Exclusions

Exclusions from a group pulmonary rehabilitation programme would include those with severe angina or signs of a recent myocardial infarction, hypertension, intermittent claudication, or

104

musculoskeletal dysfunction affecting ambulation. Malignancies affecting the cardiorespiratory system would also be contra-indications to a group programme, but individual physiotherapy assessment and advice would probably be indicated in all the above conditions.

Treatment planning

Collation of the subjective and objective findings of the assessment assists in the development of a programme for the patient which involves both individual and group activities. In discussion with the patient, realistic goals should be agreed and documented.

Individual physiotherapy treatment and advice

Physiotherapy can be considered for problems of breathlessness, excess bronchial secretions, chest wall pain of musculoskeletal origin, reduced exercise tolerance, and reduced functional ability.

Breathlessness

Breathing control consists of normal tidal breathing using the lower chest with relaxation of the upper chest and shoulders.[17] It is used to minimise the work of breathing at rest and on exertion and to reduce breathlessness. Positions that facilitate breathing control[18] and minimise the use of the accessory muscles of respiration, for example, high side lying, relaxed sitting, forward lean sitting or standing, will help to reduce breathlessness. Teaching the patient and/or the carer to position several pillows to provide comfortable support in high side lying, especially at night, can be very helpful.

Breathing control is also used to improve exercise tolerance in breathless patients when walking up slopes, hills, and stairs.[19]

Excess bronchial secretions

There are several techniques for airway clearance and some of these are suitable for patients to carry out themselves. For patients with a chronic productive cough, regular sessions of breathing exercises are necessary to minimise the possibility of chest infection and these sessions should be increased during periods of infection. Bronchodilator drugs, if prescribed, may be of benefit before the breathing exercises.

A technique supported by rigorous clinical studies is the active cycle of breathing techniques (ACBT).[17] The components of the ACBT are breathing control, thoracic expansion exercises, and the forced expiration technique. The regimen is flexible, adapted to suit the individual, and can be used for any age group and with any degree of disability. It was first documented by Thompson and Thompson in 1968.[20]

Breathing control is an essential part of the cycle to allow pauses for rest and to prevent any increase in airflow obstruction. The length of the pause is dependent on the individual patient's signs of airflow obstruction. Thoracic expansion exercises are deep breathing exercises which emphasise inspiration and use quiet, unforced expiration. Three to four thoracic expansion exercises may be combined with chest shaking or chest clapping, followed by breathing control, but it is usually unnecessary to use shaking or clapping in the clinically stable chronic patient. The forced expiration technique is one or two huffs combined with breathing control. A huff continued down to a low lung volume will help to mobilise and clear the more peripherally situated secretions. When secretions reach the larger, more proximal airways they are cleared by a huff or cough at a high lung volume. The length of the huff and force of contraction of the muscles of expiration should be altered to maximise clearance of secretions.

Studies using the ACBT have shown it to be an effective and efficient technique for the mobilisation and clearance of secretions.[21 22] It is not further improved by the addition of positive expiratory pressure (PEP),[23] the flutter,[24] or mechanical percussion.[25] Work has also shown an improvement in lung function following the instigation of the ACBT;[26] in addition, hypoxaemia is neither induced nor increased.[27]

The ACBT should never be uncomfortable or exhausting and the huff should never be violent. It can be used in any position according to the requirements of the individual. The sitting position may be indicated if secretions are minimal, but with more secretions it may be helpful to use gravity assisted positions. The effectiveness of the ACBT is dependent on adaptation in response to assessment of the individual.

Chest wall pain

Alterations in chest wall mechanics result from hyperinflation and shortening in some of the respiratory muscles. These changes can cause joint dysfunction[28] and chest wall pain[29] in patients with chronic lung disease.

Specific thoracic mobilisations, posture correction, and the stretching of muscle and ligamentous tissue can help in the treatment of these neuromuscular and skeletal changes.[30] If there is evidence of osteoporosis, care should be taken with manual therapy techniques, and acupuncture[31] or transcutaneous electrical nerve stimulation[32] may be considered.

Reduced exercise tolerance and reduced functional ability

A progressive exercise programme which would be an integral part of a pulmonary rehabilitation programme should improve exercise tolerance. In one of the few randomised controlled trials of the exercise component of pulmonary rehabilitation, beneficial effects were demonstrated in exercise endurance and self efficacy.[33] Niederman et al[34] and Menier and Talmud[35] emphasise the beneficial effects to COPD patients with widely differing degrees of severity and O'Donnell et al[36] and Rodriguez and Ilowite[1] have reported benefits in elderly patients.

Pulmonary rehabilitation programme

The physiotherapist is usually part of a multidisciplinary team which often consists of a chest physician, occupational therapist, dietitian, nurse, pharmacist, social worker, and psychologist. Programmes reported in the literature usually comprise a regular weekly or twice weekly exercise component with an educational session led by one of the team. There is variability in the length of these programmes with most ranging from six to 12 weeks.[37] Most programmes are designed for outpatients and are either hospital or community based with part of the programme to be undertaken at home. These are more cost effective than programmes conducted on a hospital inpatient basis.

The educational components

The educational components of the programme (see box) provided by members of the multidisciplinary team are outlined in chapter 10.

Practical requirements

Pulmonary rehabilitation does not require expensive equipment but the following are factors to be considered when planning the environment for an exercise programme:

- Warm, but well ventilated pleasant room
- Specified area of sufficient size to accommodate the anticipated number of patients and their relatives/carers
- Space to accommodate exercise mats during a relaxation class
- Area large enough for a walking circuit or adjacent to an area suitable for walking
- Easy access to car parking and public transport
- Availability of oxygen equipment and air compressor/nebuliser system
- Easy access to changing and toilet facilities
- Facilities for dealing with cardiac arrest
- Availability of catering facilities
- Equipment store.

Family/carer involvement

The importance of family involvement in a pulmonary rehabilitation programme has been highlighted by Gilmartin.[38] Participation in the exercise and educational components of the programme will give the relatives or carers a realistic understanding of the patient's condition and potential abilities, and minimise their anxiety and tendency to be overprotective. It is often necessary for patients to overcome their feelings of inadequacy and lack of confidence in coping with activities of daily living in the home environment. To gain maximum benefit from a pulmonary rehabilitation programme patients should be committed to continuing training for life[37] with support and encouragement from the family/carers.

The exercise component (see chapter 2)

In patients with COPD the factors limiting exercise tolerance are complex and include impaired ventilation and pulmonary mechanics, respiratory muscle fatigue, breathlessness, and poor nutritional status affecting muscle strength and endurance.[39] In patients with mild COPD exercise is usually symptom limited by lower limb muscle fatigue. In advanced COPD impaired ventilatory mechanics and breathlessness limit exercise capacity, although muscle fatigue has been shown to be an important factor in some patients.[40][41] The pathophysiology of exercise limitation has been discussed in depth in chapter 2. Owing to interaction of these multiple factors, symptom limited tolerance may be a more accurate practical guide to assessing the appropriate intensity, duration, and frequency of an exercise programme for an individual than either heart rate or maximum oxygen consumption.[42]

Blood lactate levels have been used to identify the level of training intensity, but studies have now shown that a training effect can be obtained at levels not associated with a raised blood lactate.[37] COPD patients rarely achieve their anaerobic threshold and by definition participate in low intensity training programmes. Ries[2] suggests that training could begin at a level that the patient can sustain with reasonable comfort for several minutes. From this point either the duration (endurance) or intensity (strength) can be progressed and the training intensity can be guided by use of the Borg Scale of Perceived Exertion.[43] An endurance test can be used to set the exercise prescription, for example, if a patient reaches level six on the shuttle walking test he or she would begin the walking programme at a pace equivalent to level three.

Type of exercise

Various types of exercise have been shown to induce a training effect. The most effective exercise is that which is task specific, for example, a progressive walking programme will improve patients' ability to walk increasing distances or to walk the same distance with less effort, or a progressive stair climbing exercise will improve patients' ability to climb stairs. Exercise programmes should also be situationally specific,[44] that is, directly related to the patients' ability to cope with general activities independently in their daily environment.

Lower limb activities—These can be used to train the large muscle groups. Examples of these activities are walking, treadmill walking, cycling on a bicycle ergometer, step ups, and sitting to standing/ standing to sitting exercises. Although it may be convenient to use a cycle ergometer it is not a weight bearing activity and does not involve as large a muscle mass. Cycling is not as effective in training weight bearing muscles for walking. Exercise programmes including only lower limb activities have demonstrated objective increases in the 12 minute walking test or in endurance, and subjective benefits

109

including a reduction in perceived breathlessness and an increased sense of well being.[33 45-47]

Upper limb activities—These cause distress to many patients with COPD. For a given workload upper limb work requires more energy than lower limb work and is accompanied by a higher ventilatory demand.[2] Tangri and Woolf[48] reported in 1973 that COPD patients complained of shortness of breath following simple activities of daily living such as shaving, and brushing the teeth and hair. They demonstrated shallow irregular diaphragmatic movements during these activities and deeper breaths following the activity.

Celli *et al*[49] further investigated the respiratory response to unsupported arm activity and described a "dys-synchronous breathing pattern" in the patients with severe airflow obstruction. They suggested that, during unsupported arm activity, the accessory muscles have a more active role in postural support and can contribute little to ventilation. A further study[50] demonstrated an increased metabolic demand during unsupported arm exercises.

Couser *et al*[51] found that following a training programme, including upper limb exercises (supported and unsupported), there was a reduction in metabolic and ventilatory requirements for arm elevation. Martinez *et al*[52] compared unsupported arm exercises, with and without weights, with arm exercises supported on an ergometer. The endurance training effect was greater and ventilatory requirement reduced in the patients trained with unsupported arm exercises.

Upper limb exercise can improve the strength and endurance of the muscles involved in self caring activities,[49] and it is recommended that unsupported arm activities, with and without weights, should be included in an exercise programme.[53]

Weight lifting training—Such training for specific muscles of the lower and upper limbs is recommended to be included in a pulmonary rehabilitation programme by Simpson *et al.*[54] In a controlled trial of severely diseased COPD patients, exercising three times a week for eight weeks, muscle strength increased without causing distressing breathlessness. Motivation to exercise was enhanced by patients being able to see the increase in the weights that they could lift, and responses to the CRDQ showed a significant reduction in breathlessness and improvement in "mastery" (control) of some activities of daily living.

Posture and trunk mobility exercises—These should also be included in a pulmonary rehabilitation programme. Patients with COPD have primarily an obstructive lung condition, but a restrictive element may develop as a consequence of shortening of some muscle groups and limitation in movement of the thoracic cage. Both factors contribute towards poor posture and the potential for musculoskeletal chest wall pain.

Posture and mobility exercises may help to restore a more normal posture and to reduce the stiffness of the chest wall and possibility of chest wall pain. Some postural abnormality and deformity may be a result of compensation for the underlying lung pathology. If postural abnormalities increase the work of breathing, mobilisation and gentle stretching exercises may help to reduce this effort, but there is little published work relating to this concept.[55]

Respiratory (ventilatory) muscle training devices—These have been used to increase the strength and/or endurance of the muscles of inspiration, the muscles of expiration, or both.[56-59] Training may be undertaken in the belief that it may lead to decreased breathlessness and fatigue, increased exercise ability, and improved clearance of airway secretions,[60] but has not yet been related to increases in activities in daily living and decreases in mortality and morbidity.[61 62]

In patients with severe COPD the respiratory muscles may already have been "trained" as a result of the increased work of breathing. Further training may be of limited value[59 61 63] and rest may be more appropriate for the treatment of respiratory muscle fatigue than exercise training[60]—for further discussion see chapters 3 and 11.

Dekhuijzen *et al*[64] compared a pulmonary rehabilitation programme which included inspiratory muscle training with one that comprised only pulmonary rehabilitation. They did not find any difference between the two groups in the measurements of anxiety, depression, and physical complaints.

Pursed lip breathing[65]—This is claimed to increase tidal volume and reduce respiratory rate. The technique of breathing through pursed lips and generating a small positive pressure during expiration may reduce to some extent the collapse of unstable airways, but increases the work of breathing. Many patients no longer use pursed lip breathing when they have re-learned a more normal pattern of breathing (breathing control).

111

The programme

Suggested combinations of exercise are given in chapter 10, although no regimen has yet been shown to be superior. An exercise programme should start with a "warm up" period of about five minutes of light activity of the upper and lower limbs, and stretching exercises which help to maintain flexibility of the muscles and ligaments and avoid potential injuries. The "warm up" progresses to an individualised circuit of lower limb, upper limb, and trunk exercises. Clark[66] gives two examples of possible circuit training programmes. As most exercises are carried out in the upright position blood may tend to pool in the lower half of the body if activity is stopped abruptly, and could lead to dizziness and possible faintness. A "cool down" period of light activity of the large muscle groups of the legs will assist venous return and will also help to prevent muscle soreness.

The programme should be sensitive to the needs of the individual and should include both task and situationally specific activities. Walking is probably a key activity in any pulmonary rehabilitation programme. Examples of additional activities which may be appropriate are: lifting and moving objects on and off shelves at differing heights, sitting to standing/standing to sitting and stair climbing carrying weights to simulate returning home after shopping. The supervision and support provided by a group programme instil confidence, reduce the fear of breathlessness and anxiety, and improve motivation which can be reflected in an increase in activity. Unsupervised programmes at home lack the support and interaction with other patients and staff, probably reducing adherence and may lead to a less positive outcome.[37]

Supplemental oxygen

The administration of oxygen to normoxic patients with COPD while exercising is of uncertain benefit, but supplemental oxygen is recommended during exercise for patients in whom the resting arterial oxygen tension is $6\cdot7$ kPa (50 mm Hg) or less[67] and this is discussed in chapter 7. It is not yet clear whether the training effect is influenced by oxygen therapy.[60]

Home programme and follow up

To achieve maximum benefit, exercise training and the activities learned must be continued at home both during the pulmonary rehabilitation course and on completion of the course. Training methods should therefore be adaptable to the home setting.[2] In the literature the recommended frequency of exercise activity varies from daily to three to five times per week.

Information sheets can be given to the patients after each educational session. These can act as reinforcement and can be filed in a loose leaf folder to provide a written record of the programme. The patients are encouraged to keep a diary record of their exercise programme which is reviewed at each visit. A contact telephone number for the pulmonary rehabilitation team should be available.

The frequency of follow up sessions to maximise patient benefit has not yet been identified and the requirement will probably be different for each patient. These sessions should be used to reinforce the pulmonary rehabilitation discipline and to reset objectives and goals.

Patient support groups, for example, "Breathe Easy" and "Better Breathing" can be used in the follow up component of the programme to provide peer support and social, educational, and exercise activities (see chapter 13).

Community visits or telephone follow ups by members of the team may also be appropriate. The coordinator of the pulmonary rehabilitation team should be responsible for communicating the outcome of rehabilitation and plans for continuing care to the referring doctor.

1 Rodrigues JC, Ilowite JS. Pulmonary rehabilitation in the elderly patient. *Clin Chest Med* 1993;**14**:429–36.
2 Ries AL. Position paper of the American Association of Cardiovascular and Pulmonary Rehabilitation. Scientific basis of pulmonary rehabilitation. *J Cardiopulmon Rehabil* 1990;**10**:418–41.
3 Goldstein RS, Avendano MA. Candidate evaluation. In: Casaburi R, Petty TL (eds), *Principles and practice of pulmonary rehabilitation.* Philadelphia: WB Saunders, 1993:317–21.
4 Tiep BL. Pulmonary rehabilitation program organization. In: Casaburi R, Petty TL (eds), *Principles and practice of pulmonary rehabilitation.* Philadelphia: WB Saunders, 1993:302–16.
5 Morgan MDL. Experience of using the CRQ (Chronic Respiratory Questionnaire). *Respir Med* 1991;**85**(suppl B):23–4.
6 Singh SJ, Morgan MDL, Scott S, Walters D, Hardman AE. Development of a shuttle walking test of disability in patients with chronic airways obstruction. *Thorax* 1992;**47**:1019–24.
7 Freeman W, Stableforth DE, Cayton RM, Morgan MDL. Endurance exercise capacity in adults with cystic fibrosis. *Respir Med* 1993;**87**:541–9.

8 Singh SJ, Morgan MDL, Hardman AE, Rowe C, Bardsley PA. Comparison of oxygen uptake during a conventional treadmill test and the shuttle walking test in chronic airflow limitation. *Eur Respir J* 1994;7:2016–20.

9 McGavin CR, Gupta SP, McHardy GJR. Twelve-minute walking test for assessing disability in chronic bronchitis. *BMJ* 1976;**i**:822–3.

10 Butland RJA, Pang J, Gross ER, Woodcock AA, Geddes DM. Two-, six-, and 12-minute walking tests in respiratory disease. *BMJ* 1982;**284**:1607–8.

11 Hyland ME, Bott J, Singh S, Kenyon CAP. Domains, constructs and the development of the breathing problems questionnaire. *Quality of Life Research* 1994;**3**:245–56.

12 Guyatt GH, Berman LB, Townsend M, Pugsley SO, Chambers LW. A measure of quality of life for clinical trials in chronic lung disease. *Thorax* 1987;**42**: 773–8.

13 Borg GAV. Psychophysical basis of perceived exertion. *Med Sci Sports Exerc* 1982;**14**:377–81.

14 Burdon JGW, Juniper EF, Killian KJ, Hargreave FE, Campbell EJM. The perception of breathlessness in asthma. *Am Rev Respir Dis* 1982;**126**:825–8.

15 Curtis JR, Deyo RA, Hudson LD. Health-related quality of life among patients with chronic obstructive pulmonary disease. *Thorax* 1994;**49**:162–70.

16 Jones PW, Quirk FH, Baveystock CM, Littlejohns P. A self-complete measure of health status for chronic airflow limitation. The St. George's Respiratory Questionnaire. *Am Rev Respir Dis* 1992;**145**:1321–7.

17 Webber BA, Pryor JA. Physiotherapy skills: techniques and adjuncts. In: Webber BA, Pryor JA (eds), *Physiotherapy for respiratory and cardiac problems*. Edinburgh: Churchill Livingstone, 1993:113–71.

18 Sharp JT, Drutz WS, Moisan T, Foster J, Machnach W. Postural relief of dyspnea in severe chronic obstructive pulmonary disease. *Am Rev Respir Dis* 1980;**122**:201–11.

19 Webber BA. The role of the physiotherapist in medical chest problems. *Respiratory Disease in Practice* 1991;Feb/Mar:12–15.

20 Thompson B, Thompson HT. Forced expiration exercises in asthma and their effect on FEV_1. *New Zealand Journal of Physiotherapy* 1968;**3**:19–21.

21 Pryor JA, Webber BA, Hodson ME, Batten JC. Evaluation of the forced expiration technique as an adjunct to postural drainage in treatment of cystic fibrosis. *BMJ* 1979;**2**:417–18.

22 Pryor JA, Webber BA. An evaluation of the forced expiration technique as an adjunct to postural drainage. *Physiotherapy* 1979;**65**:304–7.

23 Hofmeyr JL, Webber BA, Hodson ME. Evaluation of positive expiratory pressure as an adjunct to chest physiotherapy in the treatment of cystic fibrosis. *Thorax* 1986;**41**:951–4.

24 Pryor JA, Webber BA, Hodson ME, Warner JO. The Flutter VRP1 as an adjunct to chest physiotherapy in cystic fibrosis. *Respir Med* 1994;**88**:677–81.

25 Pryor JA, Parker RA, Webber BA. A comparison of mechanical and manual percussion as adjuncts to postural drainage in the treatment of cystic fibrosis in adolescents and adults. *Physiotherapy* 1981;**67**:140–1.

26 Webber BA, Hofmeyr JL, Morgan MDL, Hodson ME. Effects of postural drainage, incorporating the forced expiration technique, on pulmonary function in cystic fibrosis. *Br J Dis Chest* 1986;**80**:353–9.

27 Pryor JA, Webber BA, Hodson ME. Effect of chest physiotherapy on oxygen saturation in patients with cystic fibrosis. *Thorax* 1990;**45**:77.

28 Vibekk P. Chest mobilization and respiratory function. In: Pryor JA (ed), *Respiratory care*. Edinburgh: Churchill Livingstone, 1991:103–19.

29 Wyke B. The neurological basis of thoracic spinal pain. *Rheumatology and Physical Medicine* 1970;**10**:356–67.

30 Maitland GD. *Vertebral manipulation*, 5th edn. London: Butterworths, 1986.

31 Jackson DA. Acupuncture. In: Wells PE, Frampton V, Bowsher D (eds). *Pain: management and control in physiotherapy.* London: Butterworth-Heinemann, 1988:71–88.
32 Frampton V. Transcutaneous electrical nerve stimulation and chronic pain. In: Wells PE, Frampton V, Bowsher D (eds), *Pain: management and control in physiotherapy.* London: Butterworth-Heinemann, 1988:89–112.
33 Toshima MT, Kaplan RM, Ries AL. Experimental evaluation of rehabilitation in chronic obstructive pulmonary disease: short-term effects on exercise endurance and health status. *Health Psychol* 1990;9:237–52.
34 Niederman MS, Clemente PH, Fein AM, *et al.* Benefits of a multidisciplinary pulmonary rehabilitation program. *Chest* 1991;99:798–804.
35 Menier RJ, Talmud J. Benefits of a multidisciplinary pulmonary rehabilitation programme. *Chest* 1994;105:640–1.
36 O'Donnell DE, Webb KA, McGuire MA. Older patients with COPD: benefits of exercise training. *Geriatrics* 1993;48:59–66.
37 Casaburi R. Exercise training in chronic obstructive lung disease. In: Casaburi R, Petty TL (eds), *Principles and practice of pulmonary rehabilitation.* Philadelphia: WB Saunders, 1993:204–24.
38 Gilmartin ME. Patient and family education. *Clin Chest Med* 1986;7:619–27.
39 Belman MJ. Exercise in patients with chronic obstructive pulmonary disease. *Thorax* 1993;48:936–46.
40 Killian KJ, Leblanc P, Martin DH, Summers E, Jones NL, Campbell EJM. Exercise capacity and ventilatory, circulatory, and symptom limitation in patients with chronic airflow limitation. *Am Rev Respir Dis* 1992;146:935–40.
41 Rampulla C, Baiocchi S, Dacosto E, Ambrosino N. Dyspnea on exercise: pathophysiologic mechanisms. *Chest* 1992;101:248S–52S.
42 Belman MJ. Exercise in chronic obstructive pulmonary disease. *Clin Chest Med* 1986;7:585–97.
43 Chida M, Inase N, Ichioka M, Miyazato I, Marumo F. Ratings of perceived exertion in chronic obstructive pulmonary disease—a possible indicator for exercise training with this disease. *Eur J Appl Physiol* 1991;62:390–3.
44 Ojanen M, Lahdensuo A, Laitinen J, Karvonen J. Psychosocial changes in patients participating in a chronic obstructive pulmonary disease rehabilitation program. *Respiration* 1993;60:96–102.
45 Cockcroft AE, Saunders MJ, Berry G. Randomised controlled trial of rehabilitation in chronic respiratory disability. *Thorax* 1981;36:200–3.
46 McGavin CR, Gupta SP, Lloyd E, McHardy GJR. Physical rehabilitation for the chronic bronchitic: results of a controlled trial of exercises in the home. *Thorax* 1977;32:307–11.
47 Strijbos JH, Koëter GH, Meinesz AF. Home care rehabilitation and perception of dyspnea in chronic obstructive pulmonary disease (COPD) patients. *Chest* 1990;97:109S–10S.
48 Tangri S, Woolf CR. The breathing pattern in chronic obstructive lung disease during the performance of some common daily activities. *Chest* 1973;63:126–7.
49 Celli BR, Rassulo J, Make BJ. Dyssynchronous breathing during arm but not leg exercise in patients with chronic airflow obstruction. *N Engl J Med* 1986;314:1485–90.
50 Criner GJ, Celli BR. Effect of unsupported arm exercise on ventilatory muscle recruitment in patients with severe chronic airflow obstruction. *Am Rev Respir Dis* 1988;138:856–61.
51 Couser JI, Martinez FJ, Celli BR. Pulmonary rehabilitation that includes arm exercise reduces metabolic and ventilatory requirements for simple arm elevation. *Chest* 1993;103:37–41.
52 Martinez FJ, Vogel PD, Dupont DN, Stanopoulos I, Gray A, Beamis JF. Supported arm exercise vs unsupported arm exercise in the rehabilitation of patients with severe chronic airflow obstruction. *Chest* 1993;103:1397–402.

53 Celli BR. Arm exercise and ventilation. *Chest* 1988;**93**:673–4.
54 Simpson K, Killian K, McCartney N, Stubbing DG, Jones NL. Randomised controlled trial of weightlifting exercise in patients with chronic airflow limitation. *Thorax* 1992;**47**:70–5.
55 Carr L. Manual therapy for patients with respiratory disease. *Journal of the Association of Chartered Physiotherapists in Respiratory Care* 1993;**23**:13–15.
56 Leith DE, Bradley M. Ventilatory muscle strength and endurance training. *J Appl Physiol* 1976;**41**:508–16.
57 Pardy RL, Rivington RN, Despas PJ, Macklem PT. The effects of inspiratory muscle training on exercise performance in chronic airflow limitation. *Am Rev Respir Dis* 1981;**123**:426–33.
58 Pardy RL, Reid WD, Belman MJ. Respiratory muscle training. *Clin Chest Med* 1988;**9**:287–96.
59 Goldstein RS. Ventilatory muscle training. *Thorax* 1993;**48**:1025–33.
60 Donner CF, Howard P. Pulmonary rehabilitation in chronic obstructive pulmonary disease (COPD) with recommendations for its use. *Eur Respir J* 1992;**5**:266–75.
61 Pardy RL, Fairbarn MS, Blackie SP. Respiratory muscle training. *Problems in Respiratory Care* 1990;**3**:483–92.
62 Smith K, Cook D, Guyatt GH, Madhavan J, Oxman AD. Respiratory muscle training in chronic airflow limitation: meta-analysis. *Am Rev Respir Dis* 1992; **145**:533–9.
63 Moxham J. Respiratory muscle weakness—its recognition and management. *Respiratory Disease in Practice* 1991; April/May:12–17.
64 Dekhuijzen PNR, Beek MML, Folgering HTM, Van Herwaarden CLA. Psychological changes during pulmonary rehabilitation and target-flow inspiratory muscle training in COPD patients with a ventilatory limitation during exercise. *Int J Rehabil Res* 1990;**13**:109–17.
65 Mueller RE, Petty TL, Filley GF. Ventilation and arterial blood gas changes induced by pursed lips breathing. *J Appl Physiol* 1970;**28**:784–9.
66 Clark CJ. Setting up a pulmonary rehabilitation programme. *Thorax* 1994;**49**: 270–8.
67 Moser KM, Bokinsky GE, Savage RT, Archbald CJ, Hansen PR. Results of a comprehensive rehabilitation program. *Arch Intern Med* 1980;**140**:1596–601.

7 Long term domiciliary oxygen therapy in COPD

JC WATERHOUSE, MI WALTERS,
PR EDWARDS, P HOWARD

Chronic respiratory failure is a terminal event for many types of chronic respiratory disorder. Supplemental oxygen forms a fundamental part of treatment but its application is not easy and it has to be conducted for long periods of time. Long term oxygen will, of necessity, be given mostly in the home environment. It must be distinguished from short term oxygen administration for acute respiratory failure where the aims are quite different and intertwined more positively with mechanical ventilatory support.

Long term oxygen therapy (LTOT) utilises low dose supplementation of the inspired air to achieve an inspired oxygen concentration of approximately 30%. The figure was determined by early studies in chronic obstructive pulmonary disease (COPD), the most common cause of chronic respiratory failure.[1] Substantial elevation of arterial carbon dioxide tension ($Paco_2$) had to be avoided. Higher oxygen concentrations interfered adversely with ventilatory control and ventilation–perfusion relationships in the lung. Subsequently, low dose techniques have been applied to all causes of chronic respiratory failure, although this may not be appropriate optimal treatment in respiratory conditions where hypercapnia is not a problem.

Aims of long term oxygen therapy

Initial investigations into the use of LTOT tended to be by small, uncontrolled studies in patients with advanced hypoxic COPD. Typical of these were the studies by Neff and Petty[2] and Stark et al.[3] In the first, a reduction in haematocrit, pulmonary artery

117

pressure (PAP), and oedema was found together with a reduced mortality compared with historical controls. In the second, five patients with hypoxic COPD and pulmonary hypertension showed a significant reduction in PAP after 23–59 weeks of LTOT. This study also reported a reduction in residual volume, although other tests of lung function and arterial blood gases were unchanged. Morbidity was reduced as judged by a fall in number of acute admissions to hospital during the treatment period.

The results of these early studies suggested that the probable benefits of LTOT might include:

1 Reduced mortality
2 Reduced morbidity and improvement of quality of life
3 Improvement/stabilisation of abnormal physiological variables reflecting disease progression such as spirometry (FEV_1, FVC), lung volumes, residual volume (RV), total lung capacity (TLC), arterial blood gases (Pao_2, $Paco_2$), haematocrit, PAP, and pulmonary vascular resistance (PVR).

The major controlled trials aimed to assess whether these goals were more universally attainable.

Reduction in mortality

The only large, randomised, controlled study of LTOT is the British Medical Research Council trial (MRC trial).[4] Eighty seven patients with hypoxic COPD and at least one episode of peripheral oedema were randomised to receive medical treatment alone or the addition of oxygen given via nasal cannulae at a flow rate of 2 l/min or at a higher flow rate if necessary to increase Pao_2 to over 8 kPa (60 mm Hg) for at least 15 hours/day. Mortality at three years was 45·2% in the oxygen treated group and 66·7% in controls. For the men there was no survival benefit until after 500 days of LTOT when the survival curves diverged. After this, the annual mortality rate was 12% in the treated group and 29% in controls. Women showed immediate survival benefit and annual mortality rate was 36·5% in controls and 5·7% in the treated group.

In the second major trial, the Nocturnal Oxygen Therapy Trial (NOTT),[5] 203 patients with hypoxic COPD were randomised to receive either "continuous" daily oxygen treatment (mean 17·7 hours/day) or 12 hours of nocturnal treatment only. The entry criteria were similar to those of the MRC study but an episode of oedema was not essential and the patients had, on average, slightly

less advanced airway disease. Follow up was for 12 or 24 months
(mean 19·7). Mortality rate was 20·6% at 12 months and 40·8%
at 24 months in those receiving 12 hours of nocturnal treatment
compared with 11·9% and 22·4% respectively in the group given
"continuous" treatment. These differences were statistically
significant.

Improvement in mortality over longer periods has not been
shown in randomised, controlled studies. The poor prognosis
of patients with hypoxic COPD with cor pulmonale has been
documented in several papers.[6-8] In most series three year survival
rate without oxygen is 32–35%, and five year survival rate 18–37%.
These historical controls compare with predicted survival in the
above studies of 50–68% and 32–53%, respectively, at three and
five years.

Cooper et al[9] studied 72 patients having hypoxic COPD with
cor pulmonale who received LTOT according to the MRC trial
protocol for up to 12 years. Compared with historical controls,
five year survival rate was 62% but at 10 years it was only 26%.
No time lag before the onset of benefit in men was seen. This
study implied a doubling of long term surival in comparison with
historical controls. Ten year survival was low.

Using the data from these studies, attempts have been made to
identify subgroups expected to benefit most from LTOT. In the
MRC study the 500 day period of equal mortality in men was
interpreted as being due to some patients having disease so
advanced as to be unsalvageable by LTOT. The test predictor of
early mortality was a combination of raised $Pa\text{CO}_2$ and red cell mass,
but even this was poorly discriminating. The authors concluded that
the most severely affected patients were less likely to benefit from
LTOT and that early treatment should be instituted.

In the NOTT study, those subgroups with a relatively higher
$Pa\text{CO}_2$, haematocrit, PAP, systemic acidosis, and lower FVC showed
the most benefit from continuous treatment, suggesting that
maximal benefit would occur in patients with at least moderately
advanced disease. In a longer term follow up of patients in the
NOTT trial, Timms et al[10] showed that a significant fall in PAP
after six months of LTOT was associated with increased survival
at eight years.

Another claimed predictor of mortality is the response of mean
PAP to 24 hours of oxygen therapy. Ashutosh and Dunsky[11]
measured this in 43 patients with COPD who were starting LTOT.
A fall in PAP of more than 5 mm Hg was associated with a three

119

year mortality rate of 30% compared with 90% in non-responders. In the study by Cooper et al[9] survival was significantly impaired in patients started on LTOT within two months of the first episode of oedema.

Nocturnal desaturation may be important to the pathogenesis and progression of pulmonary hypertension.[12] Carrol et al[13] studied 10 patients with COPD receiving LTOT who had a resting Pao_2 of more than 8 kPa during the day while receiving oxygen. Overnight oximetry showed that four patients had significant nocturnal desaturation despite concurrent oxygen therapy. It is possible that abolishing such desaturation may result in a further improvement in survival in patients treated with LTOT.

The effect of LTOT on mortality in other pulmonary disorders has hardly been studied. There are no large controlled trials, and these are urgently required. Zinman et al[14] performed a randomised controlled trial in 28 hypoxic patients with cystic fibrosis. No effect on mortality was seen after three years. Data from the Swedish oxygen register[15] show a three year survival rate of only 22% in hypoxic patients with interstitial lung disease but 62% in hypoxic patients after tuberculosis. The nature of the underlying disease responsible for respiratory failure is clearly important; survival benefit in fibrosing alveolitis would seem unlikely.

Summary

Although there seems little doubt that LTOT is of benefit in patients with advanced hypoxic COPD, exactly how far advanced the disease needs to be for benefit to be seen is as yet unclear. Initiation of treatment at an early stage in advanced COPD seems to be important as mortality is extremely high despite LTOT in the most severely affected patients. Predictors of benefit such as changes in PAP are sufficiently interesting to require further confirmation.

Improvement in quality of life

Assessment of outcome other than by survival is difficult but is usually approached by subjective and/or objective tests of neuropsychological functioning, levels of emotional disturbance, activities of daily living, and exercise tolerance.[16]

A striking feature of most series is the very high level of emotional and mood disturbances in patients with COPD. For example, Boruk et al[17] found that, of 48 patients with severe hypoxic COPD receiving or who had been accepted for LTOT, only four had no evidence of depression and only two had a "normal" level of anxiety. Low self esteem was universal. Current work in stable COPD shows preservation of mental state.

Heaton et al[16] studied patients from the NOTT trial by means of neuropsychological testing, emotional status, and general quality of life. There was a significantly greater improvement in performance in the neuropsychological tests including simple sensory and motor ability, flexibility of thinking, and verbal/language functioning after six months of oxygen treatment compared with the findings on re-testing normal controls. These improvements were generally slight and relatively subtle, however, and ". . . did not constitute a major reversal of neuropsychological impairment in the patients with COPD". In the same study there was no evidence for LTOT causing a reduction in mood disturbance or emotional distress and no improvement in general quality of life. The authors argued that stabilisation might in itself represent a treatment success as a deterioration might have been expected to occur. No control data to support this contention were offered.

Lahdensuo et al[18] performed a similar analysis of 26 patients with severe COPD before and during LTOT for a six month period. Depression was reduced after treatment at a level approaching significance ($p<0.06$), but subjective and objective assessment of a range of activities of daily living and exercise tolerance showed no significant change.

In the MRC study[4] quality of life was not specifically assessed. There were, however, no significant differences in the number of days spent in hospital or at work in the treated and control groups. In contrast, Dilworth et al[19] studied 30 patients with mainly COPD who had recently been started on oxygen via an oxygen concentrator. Of these more than 80% reported considerable improvements in general well being and breathlessness, and more than half in exercise tolerance and sleep pattern. Control measurements were again a problem.

Although widely prescibed for palliation, benefit from the use of oxygen in interstitial lung disease, cystic fibrosis, and malignancy has rarely been studied. Zinman et al[14] performed a randomised trial of nocturnal oxygen therapy in 28 patients with advanced cystic fibrosis. No significant differences were found between control and oxygen groups in exercise tolerance, psychological status, or hospitalisation. There was a significant decrease in attendance at work or school in the control group. In this study the treated patients received oxygen for a mean of seven hours/day.

Similar studies have not been carried out in patients with interstitial lung disease or as palliation in terminally ill patients.

Improvement/stabilisation of physiological parameters

Early studies suggested that a reduction in morbidity and mortality would be achieved by preventing progression or even reversing the underlying disease process. Despite significant survival benefit, consistent improvements in physiological variables have been more difficult to demonstrate.

In the MRC study[4] surviving patients in the treatment and control groups showed no significant differences in spirometry measurements, arterial blood gas tensions, or haematocrit. There was a significant increase in PVR in the controls but not in the patients receiving LTOT, with a similar but smaller effect in PAP.

In the NOTT study[5] the only significant differences in physiological variables were a larger fall in haematocrit for the continuously treated group and a decrease in PVR compared with a slight increase in patients receiving nocturnal oxygen only. For both groups combined, the only significant changes were a fall in PVR and haematocrit after six months of treatment. The importance of these changes is unclear because, although patients with a high PVR and haematocrit had the highest mortality, the greatest benefit in increased survival was seen in patients with lower levels of PVR and haematocrit who had smaller falls in these values. There were no significant changes in mean PAP, spirometric indices, or arterial blood gas tension.

In the long term study by Cooper et al[8] there were no significant differences in mean PAP or PVR after 12 months of LTOT. Several patients were re-examined more than five years later and the stability of the pulmonary haemodynamics was confirmed. Death seemed more related to FEV_1 than to levels of blood gases or pulmonary vascular parameters.

Others have claimed a more dramatic response in physiological variables during LTOT, particularly Weitzenblum et al[20] who recorded changes in 24 patients with severe COPD in the period before (mean 53 (41) months) and during (mean 44 (30) months) LTOT. They found a significant slowing in the decline in FEV_1, a stabilisation of blood gas tensions, and a modest improvement in

122

mean PAP during the period on LTOT compared with a steady worsening of all these values before treatment.

Other reports of dramatic improvements in patients receiving LTOT have tended to be confined to treatment periods of a few weeks only. For example, Glusokowski et al[21] showed an increase in FEV_1 and FVC, together with a significant fall in mean PAP and haematocrit, in patients after six weeks of LTOT.

In other diseases the evidence for changes in physiological variables during LTOT is much more scanty. The trial by Zinman et al[14] in patients with cystic fibrosis found no significant differences in spirometric values, arterial blood gases, or maximal oxygen uptake between controls and patients during LTOT.

There is thus some evidence that progression of pulmonary hypertension may be slowed, stopped, or partially reversed by reductions in PVR. Evidence for improvements in other physiological variables is conflicting, but in most series a decline in FEV_1 continues inexorably. Even if reversal of pulmonary hypertension is confirmed, its relevance in terms of survival is not yet clear. Most of the evidence for improvements in physiological variables comes from longitudinal studies with patients acting as their own controls or by comparison with historical controls. Randomised, controlled studies are rare.

Summary

LTOT has only been shown to achieve the aim of reduced mortality in patients with advanced hypoxic COPD. Evidence for beneficial effects on quality of life and physiological parameters is scanty. The effect of increased survival has been sufficient to ensure the widespread adoption of LTOT for patients fulfilling the entry criteria. Progress with LTOT may come from a more accurate definition of those groups most likely to benefit, and a better definition of benefit other than survival. In other conditions there is an urgent need for good clinical trials to assess the effectiveness of LTOT in palliation and reducing mortality.

Criteria for LTOT

Current admission criteria

The criteria used to select patients suitable for LTOT are based on the two major trials[45] and can be summarised as follows. Non-smoking patients with stable, severe obstructive pulmonary disease ($FEV_1 < 1.5$ l) and arterial hypoxaemia ($PaO_2 < 7.3$ kPa [55 mm Hg]) with or without hypercapnia may benefit from the prescription of low flow domiciliary oxygen used in excess of 15 hours/day. These criteria have been chosen for the following reasons.

Arterial hypoxaemia

The main indication for LTOT in patients with COPD is an arterial oxygen tension of less than 7.3 kPa (55 mm Hg). This figure was selected as it marks the point on the oxyhaemoglobin dissociation curve where a significant reduction in oxygen delivery to the tissues begins to occur and further small decreases in PaO_2 result in significant increases in tissue hypoxia.

Spirometry

Spirometric analysis is an essential part of patient selection for several reasons: first, to confirm an obstructive disorder as the aetiology of the hypoxaemia rather than interstitial lung disease for which there is no controlled trial benefit of LTOT, and second, as LTOT does not halt the progressive decline in lung function or resting arterial hypoxaemia it is unlikely that patients with a very low FEV_1 (<0.6 l) will benefit as much. An FEV_1 of less than 1.5 l and FVC of less than 2 l indicate relatively severe COPD, but not severe enough to make the use of LTOT unlikely to improve survival. Predicted values for FEV_1 should, however, be borne in mind.

Disease stability

The importance of ensuring disease stability before prescribing domiciliary oxygen has been shown both in the NOTT study[5] and by Levi-Valensi et al[22] who found that, over a three month stabilisation period following an acute exacerbation of COPD, about 30% of patients improved their arterial oxygen tensions merely by optimising medical management to the extent that they no longer fulfilled the selection criteria for LTOT. For this reason both arterial hypoxaemia and spirometric values should be re-tested after an interval of at least three weeks, and perhaps up to three months after an acute exacerbation, to ensure stability. A variation of over 20% in spirometric values and a 0.6 kPa (5 mm Hg) variation in arterial hypoxaemia suggests instability and the need for continued observation rather than immediate oxygen prescription.

124

Oedema formation

Oedema is an easily recognisable clinical marker of cor pulmonale and of a clearly defined stage in the evolution of COPD. It was used as an entry criterion in the MRC trial[4] as it was thought to delineate a group likely to benefit from supplemental oxygen. Its one main disadvantage as a criterion is the link with a poor prognosis (67% five year mortality rate in the untreated group of the MRC trial).

Non-smoking

Continued cigarette smoking in patients on domiciliary oxygen not only poses a significant fire hazard but has also been shown to attenuate its benefits.[23] In some countries carboxyhaemoglobin levels are measured to assess compliance with cessation of smoking before installation of an oxygen concentrator.

Current indications in the UK

These fall into three categories:[24]

1 Absolute (hypoxaemic COPD with Pao_2 <7·3 kPa (55 mm Hg), $Paco_2$ >6·0 kPa (45 mm Hg), oedema likely, FEV_1 <1·5 l, FVC <2·0 l)
2 Relative (as in (1) but without oedema or hypercapnia)
3 Terminal (respiratory failure from any cause).

Although these three indications are also used in the United States of America,[25] a fourth group of patients is included with Pao_2 of 7·3–8·0 kPa (55–60 mm Hg), with either elevated haematocrit, elevated PAP, or evidence of cor pulmonale ("P" pulmonale—p waves taller than two small squares as a standard ECG—or oedema). Relatively few studies have been performed to support the use of the fourth criterion. The indications are based on physiological considerations and anecdotal clinical evidence. For example, although the severity of polycythaemia (an indicator of tissue hypoxia) may be related to severity of the underlying chest disease and, as such, may have prognostic implications, LTOT results in only slight falls in haematocrit.[5] On the other hand, pulmonary artery hypertension worsens prognosis[26] and those patients with the best reductions in PAP on LTOT benefit the most in terms of survival.[5]

Intercountry variation in selection criteria

Minor physiological differences between the groups of patients in the MRC and NOTT trials account for some of the differences in the indications and physiological parameters measured before the prescription of LTOT in the United Kingdom and the United States of America.

Current issues in LTOT criteria

Nocturnal oxygen desaturation

Nocturnal oxygen desaturation may occur through two separate mechanisms in patients with COPD:

1 Obstructive sleep apnoeas
2 Non-apnoeic rapid eye movement (REM) sleep desaturations.

In many cases there is a degree of overlap. Some patients with COPD without significant daytime arterial hypoxaemia ($<8\cdot0$ kPa [60 mm Hg]) have nocturnal hypoxaemia[12 27] and some also have polycythaemia, right ventricular hypertrophy, and hypercapnia which may benefit from LTOT. Evidence suggests that episodes of REM sleep associated desaturation below 85% cause no clinical harm but are currently thought to be important in the evolution of the above parameters. This is being studied further to determine the effectiveness of LTOT in the prevention of their progression but no definite benefit has yet been shown. Obstructive sleep apnoeas are more appropriately treated by nasal continuous positive airway pressure (CPAP) and medical measures such as oxygen alone, although reducing desaturation, may increase the number of apnoeic episodes.

Exercise induced hypoxaemia

Some relatively normoxaemic as well as hypoxaemic patients become profoundly hypoxaemic during exercise[28] but at present there is no evidence that LTOT provides long term benefit.

Ambulatory oxygen

Ambulatory oxygen is the provision of oxygen during walking. It is given to reduce effort induced breathlessness, extend walking distance, and permit greater use of oxygen supplementation than can be provided by static sources. The oxygen may be provided through nasal cannulae or transtracheal catheters from small portable rechargeable cylinders or by a small liquid oxygen unit filled from a liquid storage unit. Higher flow rates are required during ambulation than when the patient is resting.

There are great disputes between the United States of America and Europe as to the efficacy of ambulatory oxygen. In the United States of America any hypoxaemic individual with respiratory disease or who desaturates on exercise is claimed to benefit. Few double blind studies have been conducted. In Europe only 25% of such individuals were found to have clear benefit judged by reduced breathlessness and extended walking distance.[30–32] Liquid portable systems are preferred to gas cylinders by those showing clear benefit, but liquid oxygen is generally more expensive than concentrator oxygen. There is no indication for the widespread use of liquid oxygen for LTOT to serve the few who clearly benefit during ambulation. Special arrangements for liquid oxygen should be made.

Current usage of LTOT for COPD in the UK

The volume of oxygen supplied to patients at home increased fourfold between 1985 and 1989[33] but, despite this, a significant number of patients possibly eligible for LTOT do not receive it as shown by a 1985 community survey in Sheffield.[34] Of approximately 600 patients eligible for an oxygen concentrator in Sheffield, only about 70 had been prescribed it, indicating a large population of possibly undertreated patients. In contrast, despite the strict entry criteria, a Liverpool study of general practice[35] found that only 32 of 62 patients fulfilled the criteria and in 30 of the 62 cases LTOT had been prescribed for an inadequate time—that is, less than 15 hours/day—emphasising that underusage is often secondary to poor prescribing rather than poor compliance. In a more recent study[36] 82% of patients prescribed LTOT by hospital respiratory physicians fulfilled the criteria compared with 33% of patients prescribed by general practitioners or non-specialist physicians, indicating that a significant proportion of LTOT is being prescribed without adequate assessment. In Poland the problem of inappropriate prescription of LTOT is negligible[37] as LTOT can only be prescribed by a respiratory physician, again indicating the value of appropriate appraisal.

Domiciliary oxygen consumption is increasing annually, yet oxygen concentrators do not appear to be substituting the use of cylinders to any great extent despite the fact that concentrators would be more appropriate in many cases. This in itself presents a considerable financial burden to the National Health Service.[33] It begs the question as to why so many patients are prescribed just a few cylinders per week.

In summary, domiciliary oxygen appears to be underprescribed for appropriate cases, and in those to whom it is prescribed it is often inappropriate and for inadequate durations. The correction of these ongoing deficiencies should clearly lie with the education of those prescribing, appropriate assessment by respiratory physicians before any prescription is made, and careful monitoring thereafter.

Special situations

Lung fibrosis

There are, as yet, no randomised trials to prove the efficacy of LTOT in altering mortality in patients with lung fibrosis. The death rate in many forms of hypoxic lung fibrosis is depressingly high.[15] Oxygen may palliate dyspnoea and fatigue and it may be appropriate to prescribe oxygen for this reason to patients with end stage interstitial lung disease. Assessments of benefit will clearly have to extend beyond survival. High oxygen flow rates are often required to correct hypoxaemia and larger concentrators or two concentrators in tandem may be required.

Cystic fibrosis

A randomised trial of nocturnal oxygen[14] did not affect mortality rates, frequency of hospitalisation, or disease progression in those cystic fibrosis patients having a daytime Pao_2 of less than 7·3 kPa (55 mm Hg), and hence it is unlikely to be important in the long term management of cystic fibrosis.

Other considerations to the introduction of LTOT

Besides satisfying the physiological criteria, there are other important factors to be considered before prescription of LTOT is made. LTOT confers a considerable burden to both the patient and his or her immediate family. Their commitment and likely compliance with treatment should be carefully assessed. The fact that LTOT is used for 15 hours/day or more should be clearly conveyed to the patient, and it should be emphasised that LTOT is not for symptomatic short burst relief of dyspnoea.[38] Dyspnoea should not be equated with hypoxaemia.

Home care support and monitoring

LTOT is only one component of a comprehensive rehabilitation programme of home care for the chronic respiratory disabled patient. Monitoring of progress with spirometry and pulse oximetry are part of the package. Exercise rehabilitation, nutritional advice, physiotherapy, psychosocial support for patient and family care givers, and institutional assessment are other components. Trained respiratory care personnel should implement the service through either a broader domiciliary nursing or an independent service. Equipment supply and maintenance can be provided by private contracting companies or state purchasing authorities. The use of private contractors to provide equipment and its maintenance through a rental scheme has proved successful in the United Kingdom.

Equipment for LTOT

There are three ways of providing oxygen in the home:

1 Compressed into a cylinder
2 An oxygen concentrator
3 In liquid reservoirs.

Cylinders

Cylinders have been in existence since 1888. Originally made of heavy carbon steel, they are now supplied in light weight aluminium for domiciliary use. The size most commonly used in England is "F", holding 1360 l at 2000 psi, supplying 2 l/min oxygen for 10 hours from one cylinder. A regulating head must be fitted to the cylinder. The general practitioner may prescribe cylinders and a simple reducing valve and mask to give 2 l/min at the "medium" setting and 4 l/min at the "high" setting. No intermediates are possible. If the patient needs a more accurately controlled flowmeter or nasal cannulae, these must be supplied extra to the prescription. Portable cylinders may be filled from this stationary source, but have to be provided through the local hospital. The gas expands as it leaves the cylinder to feel cold to the patient. Many patients find this reassuring. Similar arrangements are available in many countries.

Oxygen concentrators

These machines have been commercially available for domiciliary use since 1974 and prescribable by general practitioners in the United Kingdom since 1985. Electrically powered, the concentrator takes oxygen from ambient air through two chambers containing zeolite, a substance that allows oxygen to pass through when the gas in the chamber is compressed. Two "molecular sieves" are used cyclically, allowing an uninterrupted supply of oxygen from 0·5 to 4 l/min. The lower flow rates provide the higher concentration of oxygen. In the United Kingdom the supplying company installs and maintains the machines, pays for the electricity used, and provides mask or nasal cannulae as requested. At the moment it is not possible to fill a portable supply from this system. The supply is at room temperature so patients are less aware of the sensation of receiving the treatment. They are relatively cheap to provide and maintain. Many countries have similar arrangements but the equipment is provided through alternative state or insurance organisations.

Liquid reservoirs

Containers like large vacuum flasks are installed at the patient's home and filled with liquid oxygen on a regular visit by the supplier. Flow rates from 0·25 to 8 l/min are possible. The patients may also fill a portable system from the stationary supply. This system is not available in the United Kingdom at this time. Current costs are double those of a concentrator installation because of delivery expenses. There are advantages when high flow rates or a portable system is necessary. The system must be used regularly. Oxygen is vented continuously as a means of maintaining the remaining gas liquid.

The use of liquid oxygen varies from one country to another, none being used in the United Kingdom to more extensive use in the United States of America, France, Italy, and Germany.

Cannulae and masks

There are several methods of patient–oxygen interface in current use.

Oxygen is supplied on a continuous basis. Nasal cannulae made of polyvinylchloride with proximal twin prongs to introduce gas to the nostrils are most commonly used.[39] There are few complications in practice; they keep a reasonably stable position, and nasal irritation and mucosal drying are the most common complaints. Some patients prefer masks, believing there is more benefit, particularly if they have congested or blocked nostrils or are known mouth breathers. They must be carefully selected to give 28–32% oxygen at the face.[40–41] In general masks are cumbersome and do not allow for usual eating, drinking, talking, or the wearing of spectacles. Masks are available to fit over tracheostomy tubes. When masks or cannulae are selected, the arterial blood gases achieved must be checked periodically.

Humidifiers

A humidifier attached to the oxygen source flowmeter may be supplied if nasal drying is a problem. It is usually unnecessary at flow rates between 1·5 and 2·5 l/min. Regular changing of sterile water and scrupulous hygiene must be maintained if humidification is used.

Oxygen conservation devices

These are designed to allow a supply of oxygen only during inspiration, making the supply last longer. Reservoir devices aim to fill a small chamber in the cannula at flow rates of 0·5–1·0 l/min from the source, which is then available as a bolus when the patient first inspires. The reservoir chamber is placed under the nostrils or on a pendant resting on the chest. These devices are not widely used despite potential oxygen saving.[42]

Demand oxygen delivery systems

In these systems an electronic device senses inspiratory effort, delivering the correct flow of oxygen only during inspiration. The patient must be close to the source and humidification is debarred. Monitoring devices to measure gas usage can be added.[43]

Transtracheal oxygen therapy

This is available throughout the world in specialist centres. A transcutaneous tracheal fistula is fashioned surgically through which a small cannula is inserted. Oxygen flow rate requirements are halved compared with nasal cannulae. A high level of patient education is required to keep the device clean and patent. Complications such as mucus ball formation, tracheal haemorrhage, and infection can be troublesome to the uninitiated.[44]

It is also possible to tunnel under the skin from the lateral thorax to enable the catheter to be inserted into the cervical trachea. These devices are considered more socially acceptable but few physicians allow such views to take precedence over the invasive nature of the procedure. It is also possible to supply transtracheal oxygen by a phased delivery system to allow full 24 hour oxygen for an ambulant patient. The equipment weighs 5 kg which is something of a limitation. Improved patient compliance is claimed.

Future of LTOT

Increased effectiveness of low flow oxygen, more effective home care support, and better monitoring of treatment are the three most important current issues.

Low flow oxygen improves survival in hypoxaemic patients with COPD but does not influence the natural decline of airway function or PaO_2. Better oxygenation is being approached in two ways—through additional pharmaceutical means or through non-invasive ventilatory support. Almitrine bismesylate, a chemo-receptor agonist, improves PaO_2 by an average of 1 kPa (7·5 mm Hg) above that achieved by LTOT. Side effects were a problem in early studies but are more acceptable in recent studies with lower doses.[45] Studies have still to be conducted for sufficient time to elicit survival benefits.

The issue of ventilatory support will be considered in chapter 8.

Extension of LTOT to other (hypoxic chest) diseases is debatable. Most physicians draw parallels with COPD for other causes of respiratory failure and treat accordingly. Definitive studies are yet to be performed. As the underlying mechanisms of respiratory failure differ in different diseases, caution should be exercised. Better methods of assessment other than survival are required; quality of life questionnaires being studied by a number of groups are a step in the right direction.

Home care teams supporting family carers are still poorly developed in most countries. Monitoring of treatment in the home is rarely performed on a regular basis. Most countries rely on problem solving rather than preventive monitoring.

1 Campbell EJM. A method of controlled oxygen administration which reduces the risk of carbon dioxide retention. *Lancet* 1960;**ii**:12–4.

2 Neff TA, Petty TL. Long-term continuous oxygen therapy in chronic airway obstruction: mortality in relationship to cor pulmonale, hypoxia and hypercapnia. *Ann Intern Med* 1970;**72**:621–6.

3 Stark RD, Finnegan P, Bishop JM. Long-term domiciliary oxygen in chronic bronchitis with pulmonary hypertension. *BMJ* 1973;**3**:467–70.

4 Report of the Medical Research Council Oxygen Working Party. Long-term domiciliary oxygen therapy in chronic hypoxic cor pulmonale complicating chronic bronchitis and emphysema. *Lancet* 1981;**i**:681–5.

5 Nocturnal Oxygen Therapy Trial Group. Continuous or nocturnal oxygen therapy in hypoxic chronic obstructive lung disease. *Ann Intern Med* 1980;**93**: 391–8.

6 Boushey SF, Coates EO. The prognostic value of pulmonary function tests in emphysema: with special reference to arterial blood studies. *Am Rev Respir Dis* 1964;**90**:553–63.

7 Renzetti AD, McClement JH, Litt BD. The Veteran Administration cooperative study of pulmonary function III. Mortality in relation to respiratory function in COPD. *Am J Med* 1966;**41**:115–29.

8 Ude AC, Howard P. Controlled oxygen therapy and pulmonary heart failure. *Thorax* 1971;**26**:572–8.

9 Cooper CB, Waterhouse J, Howard P. Twelve year clinical study of patients with hypoxic cor pulmonale given long term domiciliary oxygen therapy. *Thorax* 1987;**42**:105–10.

10 Timms RM, Khaja FU, William GW. The haemodynamic response to oxygen therapy in chronic obstructive pulmonary disease. *Ann Intern Med* 1985;**102**: 29–36.

11 Ashutosh K, Dunsky M. Noninvasive tests for responsiveness of pulmonary hypertension to oxygen. *Chest* 1992;**3**:393–9.

12 Fletcher EC, Miller J, Divine J, Fletcher J, Miller T. Nocturnal oxyhaemoglobulin desaturation in COPD patients with arterial oxygen tension above 60 mm Hg. *Chest* 1987;**92**:604–8.

13 Carrol N, Walshaw MS, Evans CC, Hind CRK. Nocturnal oxygen desaturation in patients using long term oxygen therapy for chronic airflow limitation. *Respir Med* 1990;**84**:199–201.

14 Zinman R, Corey M, Coates AL, et al. Nocturnal home oxygen in the treatment of hypoxemic cystic fibrosis patients. *J Pediatr* 1989;**114**:368–77.

15 Strom K, Boman G. Long-term oxygen therapy in parenchymal lung diseases—an analysis of survival. *Eur Respir J* 1993;**6**:1264–70.

16 Heaton RK, Grant I, McSweeny AJ, Adams KM, Petty TL. Psychological effect of continuous and nocturnal oxygen therapy in hypoxic chronic obstructive pulmonary disease. *Arch Intern Med* 1983;**143**:1941–7.

17 Borak J, Śliwiński P, Piasecti Z, Zieliński J. Psychological status of COPD patients on long-term oxygen therapy. *Eur Respir J* 1991;**4**:59–62.

18 Lahdensuo A, Ojanen M, Ahonen A, et al. Psychological effects of continuous oxygen therapy in hypoxaemic chronic obstructive pulmonary disease patients. *Eur Respir J* 1989;**2**:977–80.

19 Dilworth JP, Higgs CMB, Jones PA, White RJ. Acceptability of oxygen concentrators: the patient's view. *Br J Gen Pract* 1990;**40**:415–7.

20 Weitzenblum E, Oswald M, Apprill M, Ratomahars J, Kessler R. Evolution of physiological variables in patients with chronic obstructive pulmonary disease before and during long-term oxygen therapy. *Respiration* 1991;**58**:126–31.

21 Gluskowski J, Jedrzejewski-Makowska, Hawrylkiewicz I, Vetun B, Zielinski J. Effects of prolonged oxygen therapy on pulmonary hypertension and blood viscosity in patients with advanced cor pulmonale. *Respiration* 1983;**44**:177–83.

22 Levi Valensi P, Weitzenblum E, Pedinelli JL, Racineuy JL, Duwoos H. Three month follow-up of arterial blood gas determination in candidates for LTOT. *Am Rev Respir Dis* 1986;**133**:547–51.
23 Calverly PMA, Leggett RJ, McElderly L, Flenley DC. Cigarette smoking and secondary polycythaemia in hypoxic cor pulmonale. *Am Rev Respir Dis* 1982; **125**:507–10.
24 Drug Tariff. *Introduction to O_2 concentrations and to domiciliary LTOT.* Publication no. FPN 398. London: Department of Health and Social Security, 1986.
25 Pierson DJ. Clinical approach to the patient with chronic hypoxemia or cor pulmonale. In: Pierson DJ, Kacmarek RM, eds. *Foundations of respiratory care.* New York: Churchill Livingstone, 1992:699–706.
26 Weitzenblum E, Hirth C, Ducolone A, Mirhom R, Rasaholinjanahary J. Prognostic value of PAP in COPD. *Thorax* 1981;**36**:752–8.
27 Flenley DC. Sleep in COPD. *Clin Chest Med* 1985;**6**:651–61.
28 Minh V, Lee HA, Dolan GF, Light RW, Bell S, Vasquez P. Hypoxaemia during exercise in patients in COPD. *Am Rev Respir Dis* 1979;**120**:787–94.
29 Davison AC, Leach R, George RJD, Geddes DM. Supplemental oxygen and exercise ability in COPD. *Thorax* 1988;**43**:965–71.
30 Waterhouse JC, Howard P. Breathlessness and portable oxygen in chronic obstructive airways disease. *Thorax* 1983;**38**:302–6.
31 Mackeon JL, Murree-Allen K, Saunders NA. Effects of breathing supplemental oxygen before progressive exercise in patients with chronic obstructive airways disease. *Thorax* 1988;**43**:53–6.
32 Vergeret J, Brambilla C, Mournier L. Portable oxygen therapy: use and benefit in hypoxaemic COPD patients on long-term oxygen therapy. *Eur Respir J* 1989; **2**:20–5.
33 Williams B, Nichol JP. Recent trends in domiciliary oxygen in England and Wales. *Health Trends* 1991;**23**:166–7.
34 Williams BT, Nichol JP. Prevalence of hypoxic COPD with reference to LTOT. *Lancet* 1985;**ii**:369–72.
35 Walshaw M, Lim R, Evans C, Hind CRK. Prescriptions of oxygen concentrators for LTOT. Re-assessment in one district. *BMJ* 1988;**297**:1030–2.
36 Dilworth JP, Higgs CBM, Jones PA, White RJ. Prescription of oxygen concentrators: adherence to published guidelines. *Thorax* 1989;**44**:576–8.
37 Górecke D, Liwinski P, Zielinski J. Adherence to entry criteria and one year experience of LTOT in Poland. *Eur Respir J* 1992;**5**:848–52.
38 Jones MM, Harvey JE, Tattersfield AE. How patients use domiciliary oxygen. *BMJ* 1978;**1**:1397–400.
39 Gould GA, Forsyth IS, Flenley DC. Comparison of two oxygen conserving nasal prong systems and the effect of nose and mouth breathing. *Thorax* 1986; **41**:808–9.
40 Fracchia G, Torda TA. Performance of Venturi oxygen delivery devices. *Anaesth Intensive Care* 1980;**8**:426–30.
41 Goldstein RS, Young J, Rebuck AJ. Effects of breathing pattern on oxygen concentration received from standard face masks. *Lancet* 1982;**ii**:1188–90.
42 Evans TW, Waterhouse JC, Suggett AJ, Howard P. A conservation device for oxygen therapy in COPD. *Eur Respir J* 1988;**1**:959–61.
43 Winter RJD, George RJD, Moore-Gillon JC, Geddes DM. Inspiration phased oxygen delivery. *Lancet* 1984;**ii**:1371–2.
44 Christopher KL, Spotford BT, Petrum MD, McCarthy DC, Goodman JR, Petty TL. A program for transtracheal oxygen delivery. *Ann Intern Med* 1987; **107**:800–8.
45 Bardsley PA, Howard P, Tang O, *et al.* Sequential treatment with low dose almitrine bismesylate in hypoxaemic chronic obstructive airways disease. *Eur Respir J* 1992;**5**:1054–61.

8 Home mechanical ventilation

J-F MUIR

Definition and goals of home mechanical ventilation

Born during the polio epidemics of half a century ago, home mechanical ventilation (HMV) has evolved towards two distinct concepts: a life support system for patients without respiratory independence (high cervical spinal cord injury, end stage neuro-muscular disease, or chronic obstructive pulmonary disease) and elective therapy for patients with progressive chronic respiratory insufficiency (mostly restrictive chest wall or neuromuscular chronic respiratory insufficiency) which prevents acute respiratory failure, preserves function, and increases survival.[1]

Patients on HMV use their respirator intermittently (at least three hours in every 24) or continuously, with either a tracheostomy, a mouthpiece, or a face or nasal mask, or an external device such as a cuirass or poncho suit. Consequently, HMV is the longer term application of ventilatory support to patients who are no longer in acute respiratory failure, and do not need the sophistication of an intensive care unit.[1]

According to the guidelines for long term mechanical ventilation by a task force of the American College of Chest Physicians,[2] the goals of HMV should do the following:

- Extend life
- Enhance the quality of life
- Provide an environment that will enhance individual potential
- Reduce morbidity

- Improve physical and physiological function
- Be cost beneficial.

Several meetings and consensus conferences[13] have emphasised the importance of identifying the problems relative to equipment, the assessment of individual needs, appropriate levels of care, and adequate long term reimbursement—these have been treated differently in most countries.

History

There have been four main periods of development and progress of HMV in chronic respiratory insufficiency.

During 1940–50

Long term HMV was introduced into clinical practice more than half a century ago when the iron lung made survival possible for thousands of patients with poliomyelitis and other diseases associated with neuromuscular ventilatory failure. After the acute phase of the illness, the presence of severe motor damage, sometimes with total respiratory paralysis, required lifelong respiratory support compatible with home management.[4]

The 1950s

The 1950s marked a period of rapid progress in ventilator support technology, with the development of endotracheal ventilation and tracheostomy, and improved survival after acute respiratory fail-ure,[5] as reported by Robert in an important retrospective study which included patients with chronic respiratory insufficiency[6] from several causes. After the eradication of poliomyelitis, improvements in mechanical ventilation techniques were mainly concerned with managing acute respiratory failure using continuous positive pressure ventilation, although there was also interest in methods of phrenic nerve stimulation to treat patients with cervical cord injuries who were unable to achieve adequate respiratory output.[7] There was also interest in patients with chronic respiratory insufficiency resulting from conditions such as chronic obstructive pulmonary disease (COPD) and restrictive disorders such as chronic tuberculosis or chest wall deformities, in addition to those with respiratory insufficiency caused by purely neurological

136

problems. In the early 1970s[8] HMV administered via a mouthpiece or a tracheostomy (HMVT), was compared with long term oxygen therapy (LTOT) in outpatients with COPD.

The late 1970s

By the end of the 1970s, the multicentre study by the British Medical Research Council[9] confirmed the results of the Denver group,[10] showing a significant improvement of survival among patients with COPD receiving LTOT compared with a control group. Some months later the publication of the American Nocturnal Oxygen Therapy Trial (NOTT) study[11] also demonstrated a benefit for those receiving LTOT versus a control group who received oxygen therapy only at night. Those results clearly indicated the benefit of LTOT as well as introducing transtracheal oxygen therapy.[12] In parallel the important study of Anthonisen *et al*[13] on intermittent positive pressure breathing (IPPB), admittedly in less severe patients, did not demonstrate any advantage for IPPB over compressor nebulisers in outpatients with COPD.

Most recent period

During the past 10 years, interest in HMV has again increased dramatically. Several factors explain this, including advances in general respiratory care and rehabilitation, better home care services, and a new generation of compact, portable ventilators. Thus, thousands of patients around the world (mainly with a restrictive ventilatory defect) are treated at home by mechanical ventilation. A recent report indicates that about 6800 patients are receiving HMV in the United States of America.[14] In France the national association for home respiratory care (ANTADIR) manages 35 000 patients with respiratory insufficiency in their own homes and it estimated in 1996 that more than 5000 chronic ventilator assisted individuals were receiving HMV. At the end of the 1980s, a desire for non-invasive mechanical ventilation using improved types of connection devices such as nasal masks[15] increased. More recently, the use of HMV was reconsidered in patients with COPD who were severely hypoxic and hypercapnic with unstable disease which is inadequately controlled on LTOT.[16 17]

Physiological basis for chronic mechanical ventilation

Patients with restrictive lung disease

Ventilatory insufficiency with hypercapnia is met in most of the diseases associated with a deficiency of the rib cage and chest wall musculature. Frequently hypercapnia develops insidiously without any clear precipitating factor. There is a relationship between the extent of respiratory muscle weakness and the degree of hypercapnia, but the association is loose, implying that other factors such as alterations of the static mechanical properties of the respiratory system, respiratory muscle fatigue, and alterations of the central control of respiration all contribute.[18]

In chronic neuromuscular diseases, there is a reduction of the distensibility of the respiratory system secondary to the lowering of chest wall and lung compliance. This explains the resulting reduction in vital capacity, and causes an increase in the elastic work linked to breathing. It could also explain the adoption of the typical respiratory pattern of a low tidal volume and a high respiratory rate. If there is no compensatory increase in minute ventilation, hypercapnia results.

Respiratory muscle fatigue may also cause a reduction in inspiratory time and tidal volume and, if it is severe, reduce minute ventilation.[19] In chronic respiratory insufficiency secondary to muscle disease or chest deformity, the respiratory muscles may be prone to acute or chronic fatigue because their energy requirements are increased in excess of energy intake.[20]

It is also possible that hypercapnia in restrictive lung diseases is caused by an inadequate response of the respiratory centres. It is well known that nocturnal hypoventilation appears early in the natural history of the disease, before diurnal hypoventilation. Alteration of nocturnal gas exchange could progressively reduce the sensitivity of the central and peripheral chemoreceptors and thus enhance the amplitude of diurnal hypercapnia.

In most of these patients, therefore, nocturnal respiratory assistance may reduce the diurnal level of hypercapnia by several mechanisms, including an improvement of pulmonary and thoracic compliance secondary to breathing with large tidal volumes during the night, resting of the respiratory muscles,[21] and resetting the respiratory drive to a normal level secondary to correction of the nocturnal gas exchange.[22]

138

Patients with COPD

Long term mechanical ventilation causes several changes to occur in respiratory control and performance: the correction of arterial blood gases is one of the principal objectives which determines the adjustment of the settings on the respirator. HMV is preferably used at night to correct the episodes of arterial oxygen desaturation which occur during rapid eye movement (REM) sleep when the patient breathes ambient air.[23] The improvement in nocturnal Pao_2 can also increase the diurnal Pao_2,[24 25] an effect that can be related to the improvement of alveolar–arterial gradients, and to an improved level of spontaneous ventilation following mechanical ventilation. This could reflect better compliance of the chest wall and lungs, improved respiratory muscle function, increased respiratory drive, a lowering of minute oxygen consumption as a result of a decrease in the work of breathing or an increase in the efficiency of the respiratory muscles. If the cardiac output remains unaltered, then this may provide a higher Pao_2.[26]

The reduction in $Paco_2$ is also a sign of improvement in the alveolar ventilation with mechanical ventilation, which can persist temporarily after discontinuing support, and could be associated with a change in the pattern of breathing to one more favourable to alveolar ventilation.[27] The respiratory centre may recover or improve its sensitivity to CO_2, which has become blunted.[28] An increase in lung volumes (functional residual capacity or FRC and forced vital capacity or FVC) and compliance[29] in emphysematous patients could constitute a limiting factor to the efficiency of home ventilation and could even aggravate underlying disease.[20] The most important effect seems to be the reduction of respiratory muscle fatigue in emphysematous patients whose respiratory muscles become disadvantaged by the hyperinflated lungs; these patients are also subjected to an increase in respiratory work as a result of the increased resistance of the respiratory tract.[25] These results have also been obtained using nasal mask ventilation.[21] It is clear, however, that there is a balance between the potential benefit for emphysematous patients and the increase in the pulmonary inflation caused by the mechanical ventilation.[30] The long term haemodynamic effects of HMV are mainly secondary to the correction of the hypoxaemia, and the reduction of consequent pulmonary hypertension. In addition, improved function of the right ventricle can occur,[31] as well as an increase in cardiac output. Secondary polycythaemia is also controlled by the improvement of the Pao_2. The red cell mass is correlated to the mean level of Sao_2 and the lowest nocturnal Sao_2 (arterial oxygen saturation).

In patients with COPD a tracheostomy itself could be of value for several reasons:[33]

- Reduction of the anatomical dead space
- Facilitation of endotracheal aspiration and drainage
- Facilitation of endotracheal ventilation
- Possible reduction of the airway resistance with subsequent reduction in respiratory work
- Modification of FRC: as a tracheostomy makes "pursed lip" breathing no long possible, a reduction of the FRC can occur, which is also subsequent to a reduction in airway resistance
- Inhibition of obstructive apnoeas, which are present in the "overlap syndrome", that is, the association of COPD and the sleep apnoea syndrome.[34]

Selection of patients

The general condition of any potential patient for HMV must be satisfactory, with reasonably stable disease, and sufficient support available at home, to make this procedure worthwhile.[51]

Indications for HMV (Table 8.1)

Chronic respiratory insufficiency caused by restrictive lung and chest wall disorders

The best long term results (Figure 8.1)[6] have been obtained with home mechanical ventilation and tracheostomy in patients who are otherwise healthy, with disease confined to the respiratory system (often young people and/or those with slowly progressive conditions), for example, polio victims (five year survival: 95%; 10 years: 87%), chest deformities such as kyphoscoliosis, spinal cord injury, some types of neuromuscular diseases[32] (muscular dystrophy, spinal muscular atrophy, or central hypoventilation syndromes). Some other diseases are less suitable for HMV, including amyotrophic lateral sclerosis and severe interstitial lung disease. Results are similar for patients with neuromuscular and skeletal disorders with a five year survival rate of between 70% and 80%, and this is associated with a reduction in admission

140

Table 8.1 Diagnosis suitable for consideration for long term mechanical ventilation

Site or type of defect	Favourable diagnosis	Unfavourable diagnosis
Ventilatory drive	Central hypoventilation syndromes Ondine's curse Arnold–Chiari malformation	Cerebrovascular accident (stroke) Malignancy
Neural transmission to the ventilatory muscles	High cervical spinal cord injury Poliomyelitis Guillain–Barré syndrome Bilateral phrenic nerve paralysis	Amyotrophic lateral sclerosis Multiple sclerosis
Ventilatory muscles	Muscular dystrophy Congenital myopathies	
Thoracic cage	Kyphoscoliosis Post-thoracoplasty	
Lungs and airways	Bronchopulmonary dysplasia	Chronic obstructive pulmonary disease Bronchiectasis Cystic fibrosis Interstitial lung disease

After Pierson and Kacmarek.[1]

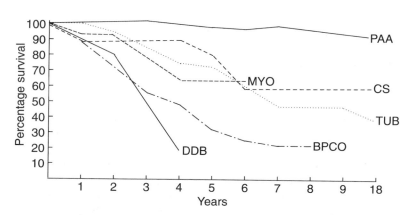

Figure 8.1 Actuarial survival of patients under home mechanical ventilation with tracheostomy (HMVT). PAA, 41 post-polio patients; MYO, 13 patients with myopathies; CS, 53 patients with kyphoscoliosis; TUB, 55 patients with sequelae of tuberculosis; BPCO, 50 patients with chronic obstructive disease; DDB, 10 patients with bronchiectasis. (Reproduced from Robert et al[6] with permission.)

141

Table 8.2 Main results of long term mechanical ventilation with tracheostomy in neuromuscular diseases

References	Treatment	No. of patients	Results (% survival)
Splaingard et al[31]	INPV	40	5 year: 76
Splaingard et al[30]	IPPV	47	3 year: 67
Robert et al[25]	IPPV	41 (polio)	5 year: 95
		13 (myopathy)	5 year: 62
Goulon et al[13]	INPV or IPPV	110	5 year: 80

INPV, intermittent negative pressure ventilation.
IPPV, intermittent positive pressure ventilation.
After Raphael et al.[32]

Table 8.3 Clinical status of 222 patients on home positive pressure ventilation via tracheostomy

	Polio	Myopathy	Kypho-scoliosis	Sequelae of tuberculosis	COPD	Bronchi-ectasis
No. of patients	41	13	53	55	50	10
Hours/day on ventilator (mean)	15	17	11	12	12	20
Frequency of suctioning (times/day)	<1	<1	4	10	15	50
Days acutely ill at home/year	7	7	13	18	23	66
Days hospitalised/year	3	7	6	8	12	22
Able to leave home >3 times/week (%)	38	—	33	24	25	0
Five year survival (%)	95	62	77	70	18	0

to hospital for respiratory failure (Table 8.2).[6] The obesity–hypoventilation syndrome[36] should respond well to HMV, but warrants further investigation.[37]

Acute on chronic respiratory failure: patients with COPD[16]

Respiratory intensive care has a major influence on the survival rates of patients with acute respiratory failure resulting from COPD.[38 39] In these patients, acute respiratory failure is caused by disease progression or an acute event such as bronchial infection, bronchospasm, pulmonary emboli, or cardiac failure associated with chronic airway obstruction.[38] There is general agreement that mechanical ventilation should be avoided in such patients with severe chronic respiratory insufficiency, because it is associated with great difficulty in weaning from mechanical ventilation.[40 41] The prognosis for those patients with COPD who survive an episode of acute respiratory failure also remains controversial.[42] Hospital mortality rates have varied from 6% to 38%,[43 44] the need for intubation from 4% to 54%[43 45 46] and the two year survival rate from 25% to 68%.[46 50] These differences in outcome may arise from variations in patient selection, and definitions of COPD[46] as well as from inconsistencies in defining the causes and severity of acute respiratory failure.[48]

In most series, COPD has been defined by clinical criteria or even by radiological signs of hyperinflation, and pulmonary function tests were not even available for all patients.[45] Asthmatic patients have not always been excluded from these studies. The precipitating cause of the acute respiratory failure is also important, because the mortality secondary to infection (20%) is very different from that occurring as a result of heart failure (40%).[47] There is also disagreement about defining the severity of acute respiratory failure, although it is generally accepted that this requires initial arterial blood gases when breathing air, with a Pao_2 of less than 7 kPa (<50 mm Hg), and a $Paco_2$ of more than 7–9 kPa (>50–70 mm Hg). Both criteria appear to be good indicators of the severity of acute respiratory failure.[43] The severity of acidosis on admission, expressed as arterial pH, correlates better with survival than does the absolute level of $Paco_2$.[49] Mortality increases markedly if the pH falls below 7.23. This is supported by other studies,[41] in which a good correlation was found between the severity of respiratory acidosis and the absolute PaO_2, and the need for ventilatory support, and an increased mortality risk.

In a retrospective study of 135 patients with COPD complicated by acute respiratory failure, who were treated primarily with controlled oxygen therapy, however, Jeffrey[51] found that the death rate increased with the age of the patient, but did not correlate with the severity of hypoxaemia on admission when the patient was breathing air, although it was significantly higher in those patients in whom the pH fell below 7·26 during controlled oxygen therapy. Age alone, however, does not seem to be a determinant of survival.[50] The influence on outcome of mechanical ventilation also remains unclear. Hudson[52] divided several series of COPD patients complicated by acute respiratory failure into two groups:

143

those treated before and those treated after 1975. The overall survival rate of patients treated before 1975 was 72%, but this increased to 91% after 1975. In a prospective study, Martin *et al*[48] found a 94% survival rate in hospital, and a 72% survival rate at two years of follow up, but he included patients who had less severe respiratory failure, including some with acute bronchitis as the only precipitating illness, in whom there was no indication for mechanical ventilation. Controversy remains, however, if we consider the series of Vandenbergh[53] who in 1968 described a survival rate of 78% with a low rate of mechanical ventilation (8%).

In contrast, Petty[10] included only patients needing respiratory assistance, and found a 76% survival rate before 1975 in contrast to 87% in those treated after 1975. Mechanical ventilation[54] itself could introduce a factor of prognostic significance. Thus, Sluiter[49] presented data which support the concept that the characteristics of patients selected for mechanical ventilation were a more important factor in determining the prognosis than the mechanical ventilation itself.

It can be seen that most patients with COPD survive an episode of acute respiratory failure, even if the subsequent prognosis for survival is poor and similar to that of other patients with COPD without an episode of acute respiratory failure.

Chronic daytime respiratory failure in COPD

Mechanical ventilation is commonly considered in severely hypoxic and hypercapnic patients with COPD who have unstable respiratory drive and abnormal blood gas tensions, leading to frequent episodes of decompensation with acute respiratory failure, in spite of using LTOT. Mechanical ventilation should be considered in the following situations.

During the acute respiratory failure episode[25 54]

There are two possible scenarios.

The patient is intubated
1 Weaning from the ventilator is possible: nasal mask ventilation may be used to facilitate the period immediately following the extubation[55] and may be continued on a long term basis if hypercapnia persists or worsens.
2 It is impossible to wean or extubate the patient: a tracheostomy

144

is often performed when difficulties arise in weaning from the ventilator, or if the period of mechanical ventilation is likely to be prolonged, for example:

(a) in patients with several previous episodes of acute respiratory failure, whose status is declining, and in whom a new episode of acute respiratory failure could be fatal (12% of cases in the ANTADIR study[56]), a tracheostomy may be maintained after the episode of acute respiratory failure with a long term mechanical ventilation;

(b) if the status of the patient is less severe, tracheostomy may be closed and followed by LTOT or nasal mask ventilation according to the level of baseline hypercapnia.

The patient is treated solely by nasal mask ventilation during the acute episode—Nasal ventilation may be maintained if the status of the patient is severe or declining. If nasal ventilation fails, a tracheostomy may be performed, followed by HMVT.

The practical disadvantages of a tracheostomy have stimulated a new interest in non-invasive techniques in these patients, such as nasal mask ventilation.[57]

At times other than an episode of respiratory failure

Nasal mask ventilation is now a possibility if the patient is worsening in spite of LTOT, and requiring admissions for decompensated respiratory failure. A European long term controlled study is being conducted to evaluate the real benefit, on a long term basis, of nasal mask ventilation versus LTOT in patients with severe COPD.[58]

Chronic severe nocturnal hypoxia

Severe nocturnal hypoxia may occur without significant day time hypoventilation in either restrictive or obstructive pulmonary disease. The symptoms are early morning headaches, tiredness, personality change, daytime sleepiness, or frequent arousals at night, and are often unrecognised.[26] Polycythaemia and pulmonary hypertension may be present by the time of diagnosis, and they provide valuable clues to the presence of nocturnal hypoxia.[32]

The overlap syndrome[34] is the combination of COPD and sleep apnoea. Relief of upper airway obstruction may be necessary, but if the hypoxia results at least in part from hypopnoeas and apnoeas, HMV should be considered. In the ANTADIR study,[56] the prognosis for overweight patients undergoing HMVT for the overlap syndrome was good. These results were confirmed in a recent multicentre study using nasal ventilation for patients with respiratory insufficiency resulting from a variety of causes.[59]

Methods

Positive pressure ventilation

HMV employs mainly intermittent positive airway pressure ventilation, which can be applied from time to time by a mask or mouthpiece, or via a tracheostomy. Intermittent positive pressure breathing (IPPB) is used for short periods using pressure cycled ventilators[60-62] for delivery of aerosolised bronchodilators. Intermittent positive pressure ventilation (IPPV) is used for longer periods of time, usually with volume cycled ventilators.[26]

IPPV/IPPB

Mouth IPPV, using volume cycled respirators, was popular in Europe in the 1970s, but it rapidly became apparent that it did not provide a real benefit for patients.[8] It differs from IPPB, in which the main role in the management of patients with chronic airflow obstruction is to administer bronchodilator medication.[26] Air compressors appear equally effective, simpler to use, and safer than IPPB, as shown in a prospective study.[13]

The major disadvantage of mouth IPPV is that it can be used for only short periods of time, up to a total of about 2–3 hours per day, because of difficulties in achieving an adequate mouth seal, particularly during sleep. Mouth IPPV can, however, be used with good results in severe neuromuscular diseases, especially spinal cord injuries.[63] The beneficial effects on arterial gases wear off after two hours.[60] The activity of the respiratory muscles persists during ventilation, even if inspiration is self triggered,[61] which explains the increase in oxygen consumption.[62] The long term effects of mouth IPPV in patients with COPD have not been documented by any study comparable to that of Anthonisen[13] for IPPB, although there are many uncontrolled or retrospective studies.[8 64]

146

In the French HMV programmes, the number of patients treated with mouth IPPV has decreased greatly in the last few years, initially with an increase in the use of tracheal ventilation[64–67] and more recently of nasal mask ventilation.[15 68]

Home mechanical ventilation via tracheostomy (HMVT)

A major feature of HMVT is the opportunity for providing long mechanical ventilation sessions, especially at night. Apart from the psychological effects, the existence of a tracheostomy reduces the resistance of the upper airways and respiratory dead space, facilitates aspiration, and alleviates some of the work of breathing.[26 33]

The disadvantage is that it is invasive, requiring more support and ideally an adherence to a general programme of rehabilitation.[14] Home care support is required and there is a significant socioeconomic cost. The risks include tracheal stenosis, although this was uncommon in a multicentre study coordinated by the ANTADIR, with 14 cases out of 256 patients with COPD.[56]

The long term results of HMVT have been evaluated by Robert,[6] who compared the outcome of different causes of chronic respiratory failure treated with HMVT. In 1973, studies[64 65] of HMVT suggested that the prognosis of COPD was worse (10 year survival: 35%) than that for patients with a restrictive chest wall or neuromuscular pathology. A more recent study by Robert et al[66] confirmed a very poor prognosis for severely disabled patients with COPD who were treated by tracheostomy and HMV, compared with patients with restrictive disorders treated by the same methods. These results must, however, also be interpreted with respect to the frequency of hospital admissions.[64 67] In a recent series reported by Robert et al,[66] (see Figure 8.1) the five year survival rate was 30%, and the 10 year survival rate 8%, for a population of 112 patients with COPD treated by HMVT.

The author's group has conducted a similar retrospective multicentre study in a large population of 259 COPD patients[56] treated with HMVT, including 58% "blue bloaters", 20% "pink puffers", and 22% intermediate type. The outcome (Figure 8.2) was a 42% five year survival rate and a 22% eight year survival rate. The survival of the patients in the author's review was better than that of the patients of the British Medical Research Council (MRC) trial[9 11] until the fourth year when their survival curves become similar. As the severity seems identical in the two studies, it seems that a more invasive approach to these patients is worth while, especially if LTOT is not successful. HMVT should therefore be reconsidered in the most severely affected COPD patients, because it may prolong survival, particularly if target levels of Sao_2 are not achieved with LTOT. HMTV may, however, be superseded by nasal mask ventilation.

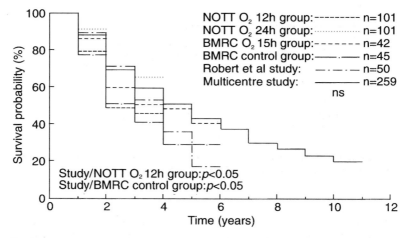

Figure 8.2   Actuarial survival of COPD patients with home mechanical ventilation with tracheostomy (HMVT): comparison between Robert's patients[6] and the retrospective series of ANTADIR with HMVT[56] named here "Study". The British MRC (BMRC) study[9] and NOTT (Nocturnal Oxygen Therapy Trial Group) study[11] results have also been reported. NOTT O_2 12 h group = oxygen therapy for 12 of 24 hours; NOTT O_2 24 h group = oxygen therapy for 24 of 24 hours; BMRC O_2 15 h group = oxygen therapy for 15 of 24 hours; control group = without oxygen. Fifty COPD patients were treated by HMVT. p = logrank test. Study/NOTT O_2 12 h group: $p < 0.05$; study/BMRC control group: $p < 0.05$. (Reproduced from Muir et al[56] with permission.)

Nasal intermittent positive pressure ventilation (NIPPV)

Initial experience with NIPPV during sleep has been promising. Improvement in ventilatory failure have been recorded particularly in patients with restrictive and neuromuscular diseases.[68] NIPPV has been intensively studied during the past five years,[57 59] with good results in acute respiratory failure,[69–72] as well as in chronic respiratory failure[59] (Figure 8.3), especially in patients with chronic restrictive respiratory insufficiency that is mainly of neuromuscular origin.[73–75] The nasal mask which is commonly used is similar to

148

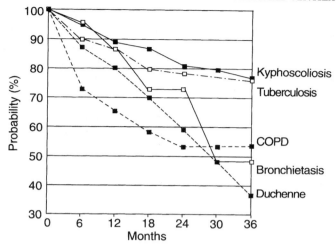

Figure 8.3   Probability of continuing nasal intermittent positive pressure ventilation. (Reproduced from Leger et al[59] with permission.)

the interfaces used to treat the sleep apnoea syndrome. In a recent study, NIPPV at night also provided good results in patients with kyphoscoliosis and lung damage resulting from tuberculosis.[15] Clearly, in patients with chest wall disease or neuromuscular disease, NIPPV improves the arterial blood gases, prolongs survival, and improves the quality of life.

Survival rates for home NIPPV are much lower for patients with chronic airflow obstruction than for those with restrictive chest wall or neuromuscular disease with a 10 year survival rate of about 10%.[64-66] Further admissions to hospital, but some improvement in right heart failure and arterial blood gases, are seen.

This type of ventilation could be indicated as a preventive treatment in severe COPD patients with fluctuating hypercapnia and episodes of acute respiratory failure, to avoid the need for a tracheostomy or to facilitate weaning.[55] NIPPV has been successfully used during episodes of acute respiratory failure in COPD,[72 76] as well as in patients with restrictive problems.[70-72] In COPD patients, however, there are few data assessing a value of NIPPV on a long term basis.[57] In an open study, 12 patients treated with NIPPV for 12 months achieved an improvement in PaO_2 and diurnal $PaCO_2$ (Figure 8.4). An increment in the total sleep time was also observed and was associated with improved sleep efficiency.[17]

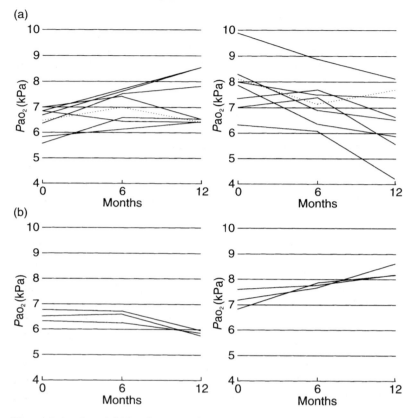

Figure 8.4   Arterial blood gas tensions during spontaneous breathing in the mid afternoon before starting nasal intermittent positive pressure ventilation and after six months and one year. (a) Seven patients still using ventilation at home after one year (——) and one patient (case 4) who discontinued ventilation after nine months (– – – –). (b) Three patients who discontinued home ventilation before six months. (Reproduced from Elliott et al[17] with permission.)

Similar results have been obtained in a recent, prospective, randomised study conducted for three months, which compared LTOT with LTOT plus nocturnal nasal mechanical ventilation using a bilevel pressure generator.[77]

NIPPV relieves upper airway obstruction and is sometimes used in sleep apnoea patients who do not tolerate nasal CPAP.[34]

In severe diffuse bronchiectasis, in which HMVT appears to be ineffective, NIPPV should be tried in spite of the high airway resistance of these patients and their considerable bronchial hypersecretion. Good results have been obtained in patients with cystic fibrosis.[78] NIPPV fails, however, to prevent worsening of chronic respiratory insufficiency in patients with Duchenne muscular dystrophy.[75]

An algorithm summarising the indications for HMVT, LTOT, and NIPPV, respectively, is shown in Figure 8.5.

Negative intermittent pressure ventilation (NPV)

NPV was introduced by Dalziel in 1832, but its real exploration began with Drinker, who built the first reliable iron lung in 1928. Emerson further improved the iron lung and it was first employed widely in the polio epidemics of 50 years ago,[79] reducing the mortality rate by 50%.[26 74] NPV has been used in other neuromuscular diseases, and has appeared of value in cases of muscular dystrophy, kyphoscoliosis, and also in patients with post-tuberculosis fibrosis.[80]

Use of NPV has recently been reconsidered for patients with COPD through new devices using light shells and jackets (poncho, wrap, or cuirass) applied around the thorax and upper abdomen.[81]

Several trials are being conducted to ascertain whether the repiratory muscles can be rested to provide a benefit to these patients. Preliminary results suggested that there might be an effect on the level of dyspnoea, on the control of diaphragmatic activity, and on respiratory muscle strength.[80–82] NPV seems better tolerated by patients with hypercapnic COPD than by those with emphysema in terms of dyspnoea levels. It is important to note, however, that a large, randomised, controlled study[83] has failed to confirm these early results.

Apparatus

Ventilators

Ventilators for IPPV are generally used for longer periods of time, often overnight. Most of them are volume cycled respirators. They should therefore be simple, reliable, portable, and easy for the patient to adjust. Both high and low pressure alarms are needed to indicate airflow obstruction, disconnection, or failure of the ventilator. These alarms must be independent of any external power source.

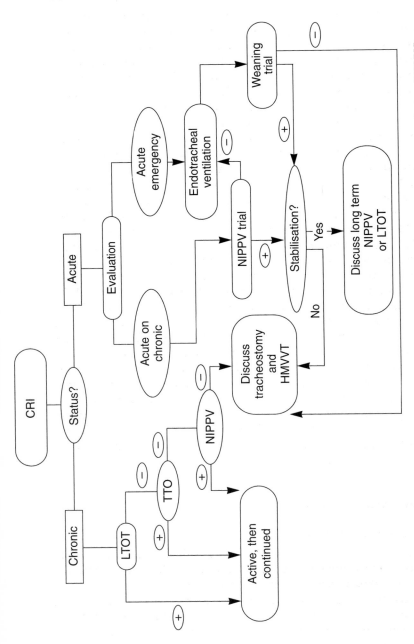

Figure 8.5 Decisions about long term oxygen therapy (LTOT), nasal intermittent positive pressure ventilation (NIPPV) versus long term home mechanical ventilation with tracheostomy (HMVT) in patients with chronic respiratory insufficiency (CRI). TTO, transtracheal oxygen therapy; +, effective therapy; −, ineffective therapy. (Reproduced from Muir[89] with permission.)

In France, several types of ventilator are commonly used, the Monnal D (CFPO) respirator remaining the most widely used. Many other IPPV ventilators are available (Figure 8.6). Negative pressure generators are also available including the Myoclet in France, the Newmarket pump in the United Kingdom, the Emerson iron lung, the Portalung, and the Life Care 170C which has recently been improved in the United States of America.

Simple patterns of ventilation are used, with controlled rather than assisted or controlled–assisted mode (tidal volume (VT): 10–15 ml/kg with a cuffed tracheostomy tube, 15–20 ml/kg using nasal mask: I/E (inspiratory and expiratory ratio): 1/2; respiratory rate (RR): 12–18 cycles/min; FIO$_2$: <35%). Supplement with oxygen can be provided by an oxygen concentrator or liquid oxygen.

Bilevel pressure preset ventilators appeared in 1990 with the BiPAP generator built by Respironics, which allows the ventilator to cycle between a preset inspiratory and expiratory airway pressure.[84] These machines provide a pressure support mode, with or without back up frequency. They are more comfortable to use for some patients than the conventional respirators, which provide NIPPV, and they can also compensate spontaneously for leaks. Bilevel pressure preset ventilator devices are under evaluation for long term use, and they may be as effective as NIPPV for several types of cardiorespiratory failure.[85] One study has produced negative results, but the severity of the COPD patients included could explain the poor tolerance of the mechanical ventilation.[86] Promising results have recently been obtained with such respirators in severe hypercapnic COPD.[77] Several new home pressure support devices are now available in Europe as O'nyx (Pierre Medical), Ventil + (SEFAM), Vential (SAIME), PB 335 (Puritan-Bennett), DP 90 (Taema) (Figure 8.7).

Connection to the respirator

Tracheostomy (Figure 8.8)

The use of a tracheostomy enables IPPV to be used for longer periods of time than with a mouth piece or mask, so that nocturnal or continuous assisted ventilation is possible.

Uncuffed or deflated tubes allow speech provided there is a speaking valve attachment,[74] which facilitates spontaneous breathing in the event of incoordination between patient and ventilator or ventilator failure, although flow of air through the

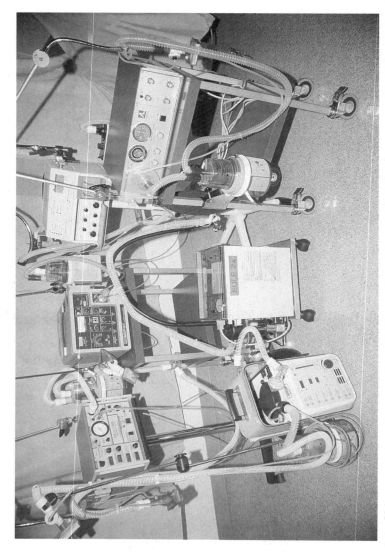

Figure 8.6   Volume cycled ventilators available in Europe (from left to right): front: Airox home (BioMS), Eole 2A (SAIME), Monnal D (CFPO); back: PLV 100 (Lifecare), Companion 2801 (Puritan-Bennett), EV 800 (Draeger).

pharynx may be uncomfortable. It is possible to achieve a sufficient improvement of arterial blood gases with an uncuffed cannula, provided that the respirator is volume cycled and can deliver about three times the volume of air that would be required using a cuffed tube.[74]

A cuffed tube is necessary if aspiration of pharyngeal secretions is a problem, or if the respiratory status and the level of compliance and airway resistance need airtight ventilation. At home, the

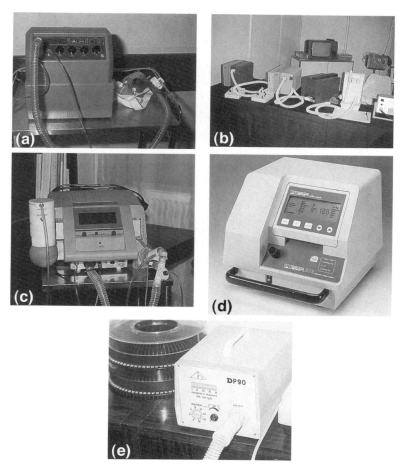

Figure 8.7 New home bilevel pressure generators: (a) O'nyx (Pierre Medical); (b) Ventil+ (SEFAM); (c) Vential (SAIME); (d) PB 335 (Puritan-Bennett); and (e) DP 90 (Taema).

155

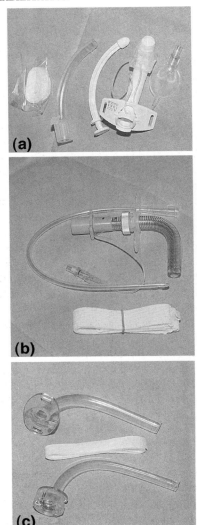

Figure 8.8 Tracheostomy cannulas: (a) Shiley (cuffed); (b) Rusch (cuffed); and (c) Trachoe (uncuffed).

presence of a cuffed tube is more difficult to manage, and must be deflated to permit speech. The patient must be educated to deflate and inflate as well as to change the tracheostomy tube, to clean it, and to suck out secretions as carefully as possible to avoid

156

tracheal irritation. Patients must be informed to ask immediately for assistance if they cannot replace the cannula because the stoma can close within hours. Conversely, difficulty in replacing a tracheostomy tube may be the first symptom of a tracheal stenosis distal to the stoma.

A silver tracheostomy tube is no longer recommended because plastic tubes are more easily available. When patients return from the intensive care unit, they are generally equipped with a cuffed tracheoestomy tube, which should be deflated as soon as possible to minimise the risk of subsequent tracheal stenosis. If the respiratory status is satisfactory, the patient can then be ventilated through a speaking tracheostomy cannula.

Humidification of the inspired air is necessary during IPPV and after tracheostomy. The presence of a tracheostomy requires suction equipment at home.

Management of a tracheostomy at home presents considerable psychological and nursing problems for both the patient and the attendant. It requires an educational and rehabilitation programme to facilitate return to home and rehabilitation of the patient.[35 87 88]

One of the goals is to have patients manage their own tracheostomy care. Modern tracheostomy tubes have an inner cannula, which should be changed and cleaned twice daily. The outer cannula needs to be changed less frequently, unless the patient produces a lot of secretions. The technique of changing the tube should be understood by the patient and relatives, but until the tracheostomy tract is fully developed the outer cannula should be removed only by experienced medical or nursing staff.

Nasal/facial mask ventilation[15]

The development of comfortable and airtight standard nasal and facial masks has enabled IPPV to be given via the nose. The same masks can be used as with nasal CPAP (Figure 8.9), but it may be often necessary to make customised nasal masks which are better tolerated by the patients and which minimise air leaks.[72] No humidification is routinely required in the breathing circuit.

From the hospital to home

A successful return home by the patient treated with HMV requires several steps.

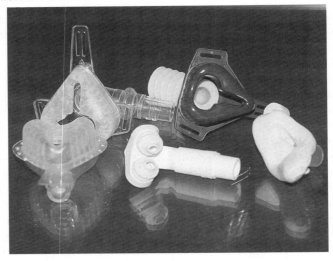

Figure 8.9   Masks for nasal ventilation. On the left: a selection of commercial masks. Far right: moulded mask.

Identifying the prime candidate for HMV

The patient must be relatively stable on a day to day basis without any gross fluctuation that necessitates inpatient care.[35] Depending on the cause of the respiratory insufficiency, two profiles can be met:[87]

1 The patient is unable to maintain adequate spontaneous ventilatory function over prolonged time periods
2 The patient has stable ventilatory failure associated with prolonged longevity, but is completely dependent on continuous ventilatory support.

In clinical practice, two distinct situations are present:

1 The patient, who has stayed in the intensive care unit, has a tracheostomy but cannot be weaned from the respiratory support
2 The patient with chronic progressive hypoxia and hypercapnia in whom non-invasive assisted ventilation might be more useful

than oxygen therapy alone. Most patients are of this type, with a slowly progressive worsening of hypercapnia and clinical status.

The home care team members

Once the physician, patient, and family have decided that a return home is feasible, an overall assessment of the patient and home is initiated, the best primary care givers being the close members of the family (Table 8.4).[87]

The professional staff involved in the continued care should include a complete team (primary physician, clinical psychologist, respiratory therapist, nurse, social service or home care planner, home care and equipment supplier) which acts in conjunction with the hospital basal team. In France, the home care service is divided into public and private organisations, the most important being the National Association for Home Care (ANTADIR), which treats

Table 8.4   Patient profile types requiring assisted ventilation in the home

	Group description	Diseases involved
Profile 1	Mainly composed of neuromuscular and thoracic wall disorders; particular stage of disease process allows patient certain periods of spontaneous breathing time during day; generally require only nocturnal mechanical support	Amyotrophic lateral sclerosis Multiple sclerosis Kyphoscoliosis and related chest wall deformities Diaphragmatic paralysis Myasthenia gravis
Profile 2	Requires continuous mechanical ventilatory support associated with long term survival rates	High spinal cord injuries Apnoeic encephalopathies Severe chronic obstructive lung disease Late stage muscular dystrophy
Profile 3	Usually returns home at request of patient and family; patient is terminal, life expectancy is short, and patient and family wish to spend remaining time at home; patients usually pose significant management problems in the home due to rapidly deteriorating condition	Lung cancer End stage chronic obstructive pulmonary disease

35 000 patients at home, and 33 regional associations which have the responsibility of LTOT (in conjunction with the private home care associations) and nearly all patients on HMV.

HMV and rehabilitation

Despite medication and respiratory assistance, many patients with severe chronic respiratory insufficiency have dyspnoea which limits their physical capacity and activities of daily living. Methods to improve the ability of patients to function at home or in the work environment with reduced symptoms (the goals of rehabilitation) have become accepted forms of treatment.[26]

The key elements of pulmonary rehabilitation[88] which will facilitate discharge should include education about the disease, the management of its therapy (that is, the HMV), physical therapy, exercise conditioning (adapted to those severely disabled patients), breathing re-training, psychosocial counselling, and vocational training.[89]

1 Pierson DJ, Kacmarek RM. Home ventilator care. In Casaburi R, Petty TL (eds), *Principles and practice of pulmonary rehabilitation*. Philadelphia: WB Saunders, 1993:508.
2 O'Donohue WJ, Giovannoni RM, Goldberg AI, *et al.* Long-term mechanical ventilation. Guidelines for management in the home and at alternate community sites. Report of the ad hoc committee, respiratory care section, ACCP. *Chest* 1986;**90**(suppl):1–37.
3 Plummer AL, O'Donohue WJ, Petty TL. Consensus conference on problems in home mechanical ventilation. *Am Rev Respir Dis* 1989;**140**:555–60.
4 Christensen MS, Kristensen HS, Hansen EL. Artificial hyperventilation during 21 years in 3 cases of complete respiratory paralysis. *Acta Med Scand* 1975;**198**:409–13.
5 Affeldt JE, Landauer K. Functional and vocational recovery in severe poliomyelitis. *Clin Orthop* 1958;**12**:16–21.
6 Robert D, Gerard M, Leger P, *et al.* Ventilation mécanique à domicile des IRC. *Rev fr mal resp* 1983;**11**:923–36.
7 Glenn WWF, Holcomb WG, Glenn JBL. Central hypoventilation: Long term assistance by radiofrequency electrophrenic respiration. *Ann Surg* 1970;**172**:755–73.
8 Levi-Valensi P (ed). *Traitement ambulatoire des insuffisants respiratoires chroniques graves.* (Colloque d'Amiens, May 1973.) Paris: Boehringer, 1973:829.
9 Report of the British Research Medical Council Working Party. Long-term domiciliary oxygen therapy in chronic hypoxic cor pulmonale complicating chronic bronchitis and emphysema. *Lancet* 1981;**i**:681–6.
10 Petty TL (ed). *Intensive and rehabilitative respiratory care,* 3rd edn. Philadelphia: Lea & Febiger, 1982:238.
11 Nocturnal Oxygen Therapy Trial Group. Continuous or nocturnal oxygen therapy in hypoxaemic COLD. *Ann Intern Med* 1980;**93**:391–8.

12 Heimlich HJ. Respiratory rehabilitation with transtracheal oxygen therapy system. *Ann Otol Rhinol Laryngol* 1982;**91**:643–7.
13 The Intermittent Positive Pressure Breathing Trial Group. Intermittent positive pressure breathing therapy of COPD. *Ann Intern Med* 1983;**99**:612–20.
14 Make BJ, Gilmartin ME. Rehabilitation and home care for ventilator-assisted individuals. *Clin Chest Med* 1986;**7**:679–91.
15 Leger P, Jennequin J, Gerard M, Robert D. Home positive pressure ventilation via nasal mask for patients with neuromuscular weakness or restrictive lung or chest wall disease. *Respir Care* 1989;**34**:73–7.
16 Muir JF, Levi-Valensi P. Should COPD patients be ventilated? *Eur J Respir Dis* 1987;**70**:135–9.
17 Elliott MW, Simonds AK, Carroll MP, Wedzicha JA, Branthwaite MA. Domiciliary nocturnal NIPPV in hypercapnic respiratory failure to COLD. *Thorax* 1992;**47**:342–8.
18 Estenne M. Pathophysiology of ventilatory failure in patients with neuromyopathies. In: Marini JJ, Roussos C (eds), *Ventilatory failure*. Berlin: Springer-Verlag, 1991:240–54.
19 Lisboa C, Moreno R, Fava M, Ferreti R, Cruze E. Inspiratory muscle function in patients with severe kyphoscoliosis. *Am Rev Respir Dis* 1985;**132**:48–52.
20 Rochester DF, Braun NMT, Laine S. Diaphragmatic energy expenditure in chronic respiratory failure. *Am J Med* 1977;**63**:223–32.
21 Carrey Z, Gottfried ST, Levy RD. Ventilatory muscle support in respiratory failure with nasal positive pressure ventilation. *Chest* 1990;**97**:150–8.
22 Goldstein RS, Molotiu N, Skrastins R, *et al.* Reversal of sleep-induced hypoventilation and chronic respiratory failure by nocturnal negative pressure ventilation in patients with restrictive ventilatory impairment. *Am Rev Respir Dis* 1987;**135**:1049–55.
23 Douglas NJ, Calverley PMA, Leggett RJE, Brash HM, Flenley DC, Brezinova V. Transient hypoxaemia during sleep in chronic bronchitis and emphysema. *Lancet* 1979;**i**:1–4.
24 Loh L. Home ventilation (editorial). *Anaesthesia* 1983;**38**:621–2.
25 Muir JF, Hermant A, Laroche D, Levi-Valensi P. Résultats à long terme de l'assistance ventilatoire intermittente chez 74 IRCO graves appareillés depuis plus d'un an. *Rev fr mal resp* 1979;**7**:421–3.
26 Kinnear WJM, Shneerson JM. Assisted ventilation at home: Is it worth considering? *Br J Dis Chest* 1985;**79**:313–51.
27 Elliott MW, Mulvey DA, Moxham J, Green M, Branthwaite MA. Domiciliary nocturnal nasal intermittent positive pressure ventilation in COPD: Mechanisms underlying changes in arterial blood gas tensions. *Eur Respir J* 1991;**4**:1044–52.
28 Fleetham JA, West P, Mezon B, Conway W, Roth T, Kryger M. Chemical control of ventilation and sleep arterial oxygen desaturation in patients with COPD. *Am Rev Respir Dis* 1980;**122**:583–9.
29 Sinha R, Bergofsky EH. Prolonged alteration of lung mechanics in kyphoscoliosis by positive pressure hyperinflation. *Am Rev Respir Dis* 1972;**106**:47–57.
30 Grassino AE, Lewinsohn GE, Tyler TM. The effects of hyperinflation of the thorax on the mechanics of breathing. *J Appl Physiol* 1973;**35**:336–42.
31 Robert D, Gerard M, Leger P. Long term IPPV at home of patients with end-stage chronic respiratory insufficiency. *Chest* 1982;**82**:258–9.
32 Raphael JC, Delattre J, Gajdos P. Indications de la ventilation à domicile dans la pathologie neuromusculaire. In: Proceedings of the third meeting of the Garches Foundation, 15–16 Nov. 1990, 1 vol, 27–38.
33 Stauffer JL, Olson DE, Petty TL. Complications and consequences of endotracheal intubation and tracheostomy. *Am J Med* 1981;**70**:65–70.
34 Flenley DC. Sleep in chronic lung disease. *Clin Chest Med* 1986;**6**:651–8.
35 Gilmartin MF. Long term mechanical ventilation outside the hospital: In: Pierson DJ, Kacmarek RM (eds), *Foundations of respiratory care*. New York: Churchill Livingstone, 1992:1307.

161

36 Burwell CS, Robin ED, Whaley RD, Bickelman AG. Extreme obesity associated with alveolar hypoventilation. A Pickwickian syndrome. *Am J Med* 1956;**21**: 811–18.

37 Bott J, Baudouin SV, Moxham J. Nasal intermittent positive pressure ventilation in the treatment of respiratory failure in obstructive sleep apnoea syndrome. *Thorax* 1991;**46(6)**:457–8.

38 Bone RC. Acute respiratory failure and COPD: Recent advances. *Med Clin North Am* 1981;**65**:563–78.

39 Rogers RM, Weiler B, Ruppenthal B. Impact of the respiratory care unit on survival of patients with acute respiratory failure. *Chest* 1972;**62**:94–7.

40 Hudson LD. Evaluation of the patient with acute respiratory failure. *Respir Care* 1983;**28**:542–52.

41 Bone RC, Pierce AK, Johnson RL. Controlled oxygen administration in acute respiratory failure in COPD. A reappraisal. *Am J Med* 1978;**65**:896–902.

42 Report of Task Force. *Epidemiology of respiratory diseases.* Division of Lung Diseases, Bethesda: NHBLI Institute, NIH Publication 81-2019, 1980:121.

43 Campbell EJM. The management of acute respiratory failure in chronic bronchitis and emphysema. *Am Rev Respir Dis* 1967;**96**:626–39.

44 Moser KM, Shibel GM, Beamon AJ. Acute respiratory failure in patients with chronic obstructive pulmonary disease. Long-term survival after treatment in an intensive care unit. *JAMA* 1973;**225**:705–7.

45 Burk RH, George RB. Acute respiratory failure in COPD. Immediate and long-term prognosis. *Arch Intern Med* 1973;**132**:865–8.

46 Asmundsson T, Kilburn KH. Survival after acute respiratory failure. *Ann Intern Med* 1974;**80**:54–7.

47 Sukumalchantra Y, Dinakara P, Williams MH Jr. Prognosis of patients with COPD after hospitalization for acute respiratory failure: A three-year follow-up study. *Am Rev Respir Dis* 1966;**93**:215–22.

48 Martin TR, Lewis SW, Albert RK. The prognosis of patients with COPD after hospitalization for acute respiratory failure. *Chest* 1982;**82**:310–14.

49 Sluiter HJ, Blokzil EJ, Vandijl W, Van Haeringen JR, Hilvering C, Steenhuis FJ. Conservative and respirator treatment of acute respiratory failure in patients with COLD. *Am Rev Respir Dis* 1972;**105**:932–43.

50 Pierson DJ, Neff TA, Petty TL. Ventilatory management of the elderly. *Geriatrics* 1973;**28**:86–95.

51 Jeffrey AA, Warren PM, Flenley DC. Acute hypercapnic respiratory failure in patients with COLD: risk factors and use of guidelines for management. *Thorax* 1992;**47**:34–40.

52 Hudson LD. Immediate and long-term sequelae of acute respiratory failure. *Respir Care* 1983;**28**:663–71.

53 Vandenbergh E, Van De Woejstijne KP, Gyselin A. Conservative treatment of acute respiratory failure in patients with COLD. *Am Rev Respir Dis* 1968;**98**: 60–9.

54 Bradley RD, Spencer GT, Semple SJG. Tracheostomy and artificial ventilation in the treatment of acute exacerbations of chronic lung disease. A study in twenty-nine patients. *Lancet* 1964;**i**:854–9.

55 Udwadia ZF, Santis GK, Steven MH, Simonds AK. Nasal ventilation to facilitate weaning in patients with chronic respiratory insufficiency. *Thorax* 1992; **47**:715–18.

56 Muir JF, Girault C, Cardinaud JP, Polu JM and the French Cooperative Group. Survival and long-term follow-up of tracheostomized patients with COPD treated by home mechanical ventilation. A Multicenter French study in 259 patients. *Chest* 1994;**106**:201–9.

57 Hill NS. Non invasive ventilation: Does it work, for whom, and how? *Am Rev Respir Dis* 1993;**147**:1050–5.

58 Morgan MDL. Conference Report: Second International Conference on Advances in Pulmonary Rehabilitation and Management of Chronic Respiratory Failure, Venice, 4–7 November 1992. *Thorax* 1993;**48**:296–7.

59 Leger P, Bedicam JM, Cornette A, *et al*. Nasal intermittent positive pressure ventilation: Long-term follow-up in patients with severe chronic respiratory insufficiency. *Chest* 1994;**105**:100–5.

60 Birnbaum ML, Cree EM, Rasmussen H. Effects of IPPB on emphysematous patients. *Am J Med* 1966;**41**:551–61.

61 Kamat SR, Dulfano MJ, Segal MS. The effects of IPPB with compressed air in patients with severe chronic non-specific obstructive pulmonary disease. *Am Rev Respir Dis* 1962;**86**:360–80.

62 Sukumalchantra Y, Park SS, William MH. The effects of IPPB in acute respiratory failure. *Am Rev Respir Dis* 1965;**92**:885–93.

63 Bach JR, Alba AS. Non invasive options for ventilatory support of the traumatic high level quadriplegic. *Chest* 1990;**98**:613–19.

64 Achard J, Alquier P, Chennebault JM. Experience de 9 années de VAD chez de grands handicapés respiratoires. *Rev fr mal resp* 1979;**7**:424–6.

65 Bolot JF, Robert D, Chemorin B. Die hausliche assistierte Beatmung durch Tracheotomie bei chronischer Ateminsuffizienz. *Munch Med Wochenschr* 1977;**119**:1641–6.

66 Robert D, Leger P, Salamand J, Gaussorgue P, Buffat J, Jennequin J. Home mechanical ventilator dependent patients. International Conference on Pulmonary rehabilitation and HMV. Denver, March 1988. Proceedings.

67 Sivak ED, Cordasco EM, Gipson WT, Stelmak K. Clinical considerations in the implementation of home care ventilation. *Cleve Clin Q* 1983;**50**:219–25.

68 Rideau Y, Jankowski LW, Grellet J. Management of respiratory neuromuscular weakness. *Muscle Nerve* 1988;**11**:407–8.

69 Brochard L, Isabey D, Piquet J. Reversal of acute exacerbations of chronic obstructive pulmonary disease by inspiratory assistance with a face mask. *N Engl J Med* 1990;**323**:1523–30.

70 Meduri GV, Conoscenti CC, Menashe P, Nair S. Non invasive face mask ventilation in patients with acute respiratory failure. *Chest* 1989;**95**:865–70.

71 Benhamou D, Girault C, Faure C, Portier F, Muir JF. Nasal mask ventilation in acute hypercapnic respiratory failure: experience in elderly patients. *Chest* 1992;**102**:912–17.

72 Leger P, Jennequin J, Gaussorgue D, Robert D. Acute respiratory failure in COPD patients treated by home IPPV via nasal mask (abstract). *Eur Respir J* 1989;**3**:683S.

73 Bach JR, Alba AS. Management of chronic alveolar hypoventilation by nasal ventilation. *Chest* 1990;**97**:52–7.

74 Shneerson J. In *Disorders of ventilation*. Oxford: Blackwell 1988:389.

75 Raphael TC, Chevret S, Chastang C, Bouvet F. Home mechanical ventilation in Duchenne's muscular dystrophy: In search of a therapeutic strategy. *Eur Respir Rev* 1993;**3**:270–4.

76 Bott J, Carroll MP, Conway JH, *et al*. Randomised controlled trial of nasal ventilation in acute respiratory failure due to chronic obstructive airways disease. *Lancet* 1993;**341**:1555–7.

77 Meecham-Jones, Jones PW, Paul EA, Wedzicha JA. Randomised controlled trial of nasal positive pressure ventilation plus LTOT compared to LTOT alone: Effect on blood gases and quality of life. *Am J Respir Crit Care Med* 1996 (in press).

78 Piper AJ, Parker S, Torzillo PJ, Sullivan CE, Bye PTP. Nocturnal NIPPV stabilizes patients with cystic fibrosis and hypercapnic respiratory failure. *Chest* 1992;**102**:846–50.

79 Hill NS. Clinical applications of body ventilators. *Chest* 1986;**90**:897–905.

80 Shneerson JM. Non invasive and domiciliary ventilation: Negative pressure techniques. *Thorax* 1991;**46**:131–5.
81 Milane J, Bertrand A. Indications de la ventilation par prothèse extra-thoracique. *Bull Eur Physiopathol Respir* 1986;**22**(suppl 9):37S–40S.
82 Braun NMT. Intermittent mechanical ventilation. *Clin Chest Med* 1988;**9**: 153–62.
83 Shapiro SH, Ernst P, Gray-Donald K, *et al.* Effects of negative pressure ventilation in chronic obstructive pulmonary disease. *Lancet* 1992;**340**:1425–9.
84 Sanders MH, Kern N. Obstructive sleep apnea treated by independently adjusted inspiratory and expiratory positive airway pressure via nasal mask. *Chest* 1990;**98**:317–41.
85 Wedzicha D. Comparison of bi-level continuous positive airway pressure versus nasal intermittent positive pressure ventilation in chronic respiratory insufficiency. *Eur Respir J* 1992;**4**:A313.
86 Strumpf DA, Millman RP, Carlisle CC, *et al.* Nocturnal positive pressure ventilation via nasal mask in patients with severe chronic obstructive pulmonary disease. *Am Rev Respir Dis* 1991;**144**:1234–9.
87 Lucas J. Home ventilator care. In: O'Ryan JA, Burns DG (eds), *Pulmonary rehabilitation: from hospital to home.* Chicago: Year Book Medical Publishers, 1984:260.
88 Make BJ. Pulmonary rehabilitation: Myth or reality? *Clin Chest Med* 1986;**7**: 519–40.
89 Muir JF. Home mechanical ventilation in patients with COPD. *Eur Respir J* 1991;**1**:550–62.

9 Health related quality of life among patients with COPD

J RANDALL CURTIS, RICHARD A DEYO,
LEONARD D HUDSON

Chronic obstructive pulmonary disease (COPD) is a leading cause of morbidity and mortality in industrialised nations. It is essentially incurable and, for many, inexorably progressive; health care providers spend much effort trying to minimise patients' symptoms and to improve their ability to function in day-to-day life. Although improved survival time is an important aim of treatment, there is growing recognition that improving the quantity of an individual's life may not be the only goal; for some, improving the quality of life may be far more important. As reducing symptoms, increasing function, and improving the quality of life are central therapeutic goals for patients with COPD, as for many chronic diseases, it is important for researchers and clinicians to develop a common understanding of what is meant by these phrases and how these concepts can be measured.

In the past 10 years there has been an increasing body of literature on measurement of quality of life in patients with COPD and, more recently, on the efficacy of therapeutic agents based on quality of life measures. Studies measuring the quality of life in these patients appeared in the mid-1980s[1-6] when quality of life measures were used to assess continuous oxygen therapy,[5] intermittent positive pressure breathing,[6] and, more recently, in the assessment of theophylline,[7] inhaled bronchodilators,[8] home respiratory nursing care,[9] and pulmonary rehabilitation programmes.[10 11]

This chapter reviews quality of life measures in patients with COPD with the emphasis on issues important to the clinician who seeks an understanding of quality of life measures as they are used in therapeutic trials.

Definition and relevance of health related quality of life

Terms and definitions

The term "quality of life" is widely used in clinical research and clinical care, but rarely defined. In its broadest definition the quality of an individual's life is strongly influenced by factors that health care does not directly affect, including financial status, housing, employment, and social support. Consequently many researchers favour the more restrictive terms "health related quality of life" (HRQL) or "functional status" to mean the quality of life as it is affected by health status. Functional status connotes a stronger basis in ability to perform the tasks of daily life, whereas HRQL connotes the subjective experience of the impact of health on the quality of one's life. As COPD is a disease often affecting older, retired persons, the mechanics of task performance may be less important than the ability to enjoy life. The term HRQL will therefore be used.

In general, HRQL measures the impact of an individual's health on his or her ability to perform and enjoy the activities of daily life. HRQL instruments vary from disease specific measures of a single (usually crucial) symptom such as dyspnoea,[3] to a generic global assessment of many facets which may include emotional functioning (mood changes and other psychiatric symptoms), social role functioning (employment, home management, and social or family relationships), activities of daily living (self care skills and mobility), and the ability to enjoy activities (hobbies and recreation).[1]

The operational definition of HRQL also varies somewhat depending on its use. In general, outcome measures can have at least three purposes: discriminating between subjects at a single point in time, predicting prognosis, or evaluating changes within a given subject over time. Although the purpose does not alter development and application of many physiological measures, the design of HRQL measures may vary substantially depending on the intended purpose.[12] To discriminate between a group of subjects, questionnaire items are selected to represent important components

166

of HRQL which are applicable to as many individuals as possible. In contrast, for use in a therapeutic trial the instrument should detect change over time in an individual, and therefore questionnaire items are chosen only if they reflect features amenable to change. An example from the sickness impact profile was chosen by Deyo in a recent review to illustrate this point.[13] A positive response to the statement "I have attempted suicide" would indicate a high level of emotional distress and help discriminate among individuals. However, the response would remain positive at subsequent testing and consequently would not help to distinguish change over time. In contrast, the number of stairs that an individual can climb might be an effective gauge of change over time, but would not be a useful discriminative tool in a group of older adults who have made environmental changes to avoid stairs.

Relevance and usefulness of HRQL

A common criticism of HRQL is that it is highly subjective and therefore inherently immeasurable or, at best, "soft" data. It is axiomatic that HRQL is subjective, because it is the individual patient's perspective that is the most important measure of HRQL. Is this subjective quality necessarily immeasurable or "soft"? As Feinstein argues, the crucial attribute of "hardness" is the reproducibility of a measure.[14] HRQL measures *are* able to provide adequate and often excellent reproducibility. If "hard" physiological measures accurately reflected HRQL, it could be argued that HRQL measures are unnecessary. Physiological measures such as pulmonary function and exercise tolerance do not, however, correlate strongly with measures of HRQL.[13 15 16]

HRQL should not be measured in every therapeutic trial or longitudinal survey. There are circumstances where survival is the paramount outcome measure and HRQL is irrelevant. An example would be a randomised controlled trial of corticosteroids in COPD patients with acute respiratory failure. This short term treatment is designed to improve survival or shorten the course of the acute illness: HRQL is less important in judging efficacy. In other instances treatment may be applied to asymptomatic adults to prevent progressive disease, such as a trial of smoking cessation techniques. In this case HRQL would not be expected to vary (or could be temporarily worse in those who stop smoking) and the benefit would be more appropriately shown in terms of smoking cessation success rates.

167

The phase of treatment development should also be considered before assessing HRQL as an outcome measure. Phase I trials are primarily concerned with pharmacokinetics and dose finding, and HRQL measures would not be appropriate. In small, early phase II trials HRQL would be unlikely to show either benefit or lack of benefit. It is the large phase III trials, especially those designed to mimic clinical practice (known as "effectiveness" trials), where HRQL can add the patient's view to other, more traditional, outcome measures.

Finally, HRQL measures can be especially useful in trials designed to assess treatments which differ dramatically in cost, side effects, or degree of invasiveness. For instance, in trials of extensive pulmonary rehabilitation or even lung transplantation, HRQL would be an important component to factor into cost effectiveness analyses.

Measurement issues

Generic versus disease specific measures

HRQL instruments may be designed to assess overall quality of life, or only those aspects directly related to a particular disease. For instance, COPD specific instruments can assess a single symptom such as dyspnoea.[3] They could also measure a series of symptoms—for example, dyspnoea, cough, and sputum production—plus those components of life particularly affected by COPD—for example, exercise tolerance and mood.[4] Generic instruments also represent a spectrum of questions and symptoms and are often divided into sections devoted to several parameters, such as physical discomfort, role functioning, emotional well being, and social interactions. In addition, generic HRQL instruments may include a summary score allowing investigators to assign a single number to overall HRQL and use this score for cost effectiveness analyses.

Disease specific and generic instruments each have their advantages and disadvantages.[17 18] The choice of the type of instrument depends on the question being asked. Disease specific instruments are likely to be more sensitive to small changes in a therapeutic trial of an agent targeted at the specific symptoms of COPD. For instance, an instrument to measure dyspnoea is more likely to show a benefit of bronchodilators than a generic HRQL

168

instrument.[18] In addition, disease specific instruments relate closely to the clinical history obtained by clinicians and, consequently, may be more readily understandable to the clinician.

Generic instruments have the advantage of being thoroughly tested in various clinical settings and populations. The breadth of HRQL issues that they cover may reveal important, but unexpected, impacts of the treatment. In addition, they are more likely appropriately to weigh diverse side effects of treatment and establish an overall assessment of treatment on the patient's life. Finally, generic instruments are necessary if one wishes to compare the HRQL benefits of interventions for widely disparate conditions— for example, is lung transplantation as effective as kidney transplantation?

Reproducibility, validity, and responsiveness

Three features of a questionnaire are important for clinicians to understand before assessing evidence based on HRQL instruments. The first is the reproducibility (or reliability) of the instrument—that is, whether it is resilient to confounding variations in the environment. There are various components to reproducibility, including test–re-test reproducibility (how vulnerable the instrument is to unimportant day-to-day variations in the subject's response), interobserver reproducibility (whether different administrators of the instrument get the same results from the same individual), and internal consistency (whether different parts of the instrument give consistent results). These issues are not necessarily re-examined with each study using the instrument, but a reader should be convinced that this assessment has been done and that the instrument fulfils the basic measurement expectations.

Validity is a more difficult issue to assess in HRQL. Validity asks whether the instrument is really measuring the impact of health on an individual's quality of life. For HRQL there is no reference standard to measure the instrument against and consequently correlations with biological indicators of disease such as FEV_1 and exercise tolerance, and other HRQL instruments, must be used as proxies for a "gold standard". Very high correlations would not be expected as the intention is not to duplicate these other measures, but the instrument should correlate in the expected direction with markers of disease severity and with other HRQL instruments. This process is known as "construct validation" and is an ongoing process as no single critical observation can definitively establish validity, which contrasts with "criterion validity" in which a true "gold standard" exists. Some of these correlations should be provided with the use of an instrument in a clinical trial to confirm that it is valid for the population under study.

For clinical trials or other longitudinal studies responsiveness is a key feature of HRQL instruments as the instruments need to identify small, but clinically important, changes over time. This sensitivity is central to the use of HRQL instruments in clinical trials to show a benefit (or lack of benefit). Investigators should therefore define the minimal clinically important difference that can be detected by the instrument.[19] Conversely, a large controlled trial might easily be able to identify statistically significant differences in HRQL which are clinically irrelevant—for example, a statistically significant improvement in FEV_1 of 10 ml from a large study would be interpreted by clinicians as clinically unimportant. With HRQL measures, however, it is usually the responsibility of the researchers to identify the minimal clinically important difference.

Statistical issues

It is important to identify the key hypotheses before data collection and to report when hypotheses were generated by analysis of associations in the data. This is particularly important in HRQL because these instruments often have multiple components and are conducive to "data torturing".[20] If post hoc analyses are performed, the level of statistical significance should be adjusted appropriately to compensate for the problems of multiple comparisons.[21]

Sample size and power calculations are important in trials using HRQL instruments because the relative inexperience of using these measures may make it difficult to estimate a clinically important difference, a central component of these calculations. The difficulty with power calculations is usually considered to be the problem of the researcher, not the clinician. In a trial showing no benefit of treatment, however, the power of the trial to identify a benefit becomes of foremost interest to the clinician trying to decide whether to abandon this treatment. If power calculations are unreliable, it becomes difficult to judge the value of the trial.

Selected HRQL instruments

There are four generic HRQL instruments and four disease specific instruments that have been used extensively in patients with COPD. Some important features of each of these instruments are shown in Table 9.1.

Generic HRQL instruments

The generic HRQL instrument which has been used most extensively in patients with COPD is the sickness impact profile (SIP). This comprehensive, 136 item, self administered questionnaire was developed to measure HRQL in a wide variety of chronic diseases. The instrument assesses a broad range of areas including ambulation, body care, mobility, emotional behaviour, social behaviour, work, sleep, eating, home management, and recreational activities. It is one of the longest instruments, requiring 20–30 minutes to complete. It has undergone extensive testing to establish its reproducibility and validity,[22] although its responsiveness has been questioned in patients with COPD.[18] The SIP has been used extensively to document descriptively the HRQL in patients with COPD.[13 23 24] It has also been used in patients with COPD to assess the value of continuous oxygen therapy,[5] antidepressant therapy,[25] home respiratory nursing care,[9] and intermittent positive pressure breathing.[6]

A similar generic instrument was developed for the Medical Outcome Study (MOS), a physicians' office based, cross sectional study of 9385 adults.[26] An initially large number of questions was reduced to a 20 item, self administered instrument divided into two parts. The first examines physical functioning, role functioning, and social functioning, and the second examines mental health, health perceptions, and bodily pain. This instrument requires about three minutes to complete and was shown to be reproducible and valid.[26] COPD was one of the diseases examined in this survey, and, although a new instrument, it has been used to assess the HRQL of patients with COPD.[27] The MOS has the advantage of brevity but, like the SIP, responsiveness in patients with COPD has not yet been thoroughly examined. Recently the authors of the MOS instrument have prepared a 36 item "short form" known as the MOS SF-36.[28] This generic health status instrument is being widely used and has been adopted by a number of researchers and

171

Table 9.1 Selected HRQL instruments used in patients with COPD

Instrument	Domains and dimensions examined	Length	Administration	Reproducible, valid, and responsive
Generic:				
Sickness Impact Profile (SIP)	Physical: ambulation, mobility, body care. Social: general well being, work/social role performance, social support and participation, global social function, personal relationships, and global emotional functioning	136 items (30 min)	Self administered	Reproducibility, validity, and responsiveness well demonstrated
Medical Outcomes Study (MOS)	Functioning: physical, role, and social. Well being: mental health, health perceptions, and bodily pain	20 items (3 min)	Self administered	Reproducibility and validity well demonstrated; responsiveness in COPD not well studied
Quality of Well Being (QWB)	Mobility: access to modes of transportation. Physical: limits to activity. Social: limits to activity. Symptoms: review of systems	50 items (12 min)	Trained interviewer administered	Reproducible and valid; responsiveness in COPD not well demonstrated
Nottingham Health Profile (NHP)	Health: energy, pain, emotional reactions, sleep, social isolation, physical mobility. Life functioning: employment, relationships, personal life, sex, hobbies, vacations, housework	45 items (10 min)	Self administered	Reproducible and valid; responsiveness in COPD not well demonstrated

Table 9.1 *continued*

COPD specific:				
Chronic Respiratory Disease Questionnaire (CRDQ)	Dyspnoea, fatigue, mastery over disease, emotional dysfunction	20 items (20 min)	Trained interviewer administered	Reproducibility, validity, and responsiveness well demonstrated
St George's Respiratory Questionnaire (SGRQ)	Symptoms: cough, sputum, wheeze, breathlessness. Activity: physical functioning, housework, hobbies. Impact on daily life: social and emotional impact	76 items (8–10 min)	Self administered	Reproducibility, validity, and responsiveness well demonstrated
Oxygen Cost Diagram (OCD)	Single vertical line to be marked in location to indicate degree of disability caused by dyspnoea	1 item (<5 min)	Self administered	Intermediate reproducibility and validity. Not as responsive as SGRQ
Baseline Dyspnoea Index (BDI)	Functional impairment, magnitude of task evoking dyspnoea, magnitude of effort evoking dyspnoea	3 indices with four grades (<5 min)	Trained interviewer administered	Reproducibility, validity, and responsiveness well demonstrated

173

health care organisations. Its validity has been demonstrated in many diseases,[30] including COPD.[30]

The quality of well being (QWB) is a 50 item interviewer administered questionnaire developed as a subcomponent of a larger health outcomes measure, the health status index.[31] The QWB is divided into three scales—mobility, physical activity, and social activity. The QWB score is expressed as the value that subjects associate with a particular combination of function and symptoms, so it can be used for quantitative assessment and cost effectiveness analysis. It has been shown to be reproducible and valid[32 33] and has been used to describe HRQL in patients with COPD.[34] In addition, the QWB has been used to assess home respiratory nursing care[9] and pulmonary rehabilitation programmes[10 11] for individuals with COPD. Although the QWB does not assess as many domains as the SIP or the MOS, it has the unique advantage of being applicable to cost effectiveness analysis.

Finally, the Nottingham health profile (NHP) is a 45 item, self administered questionnaire composed of two parts. The first contains 38 items assessing energy, pain, emotional reactions, sleep, social isolation, and physical mobility, and the second part contains seven items covering the areas of life functioning most often affected by health problems. This self administered instrument takes 10 minutes to complete. It is reproducible and valid in the assessment of chronic diseases[35] and has been used to describe HRQL in patients with COPD.[36] The NHP has recently been used to assess inhaled bronchodilators in patients with COPD.[37]

Several other instruments which measure mood, depression, anxiety, and other psychiatric symptoms have been used to assess patients with COPD. These include the Minnesota Multiphasic Personality Inventory (MMPI), the Profile of Mood States (POMS), and the Beck Depression Inventory.[12 26 38] Although these instruments have provided insights into the HRQL of persons with COPD and may provide important information in the assessment of treatment for COPD, they are not strictly measures of HRQL and will not be discussed in detail in this chapter.

Disease specific HRQL instruments

The Chronic Respiratory Disease Questionnaire (CRDQ) was developed by Guyatt and colleagues through in-depth, unstructured

174

interviews in 100 patients with COPD. The result was a 20 item questionnaire dealing with dimensions of dyspnoea, fatigue, patients' sense of control over the disease (mastery), and emotional dysfunction. This interviewer administered questionnaire takes 20 minutes to complete and has been shown to be reproducible, valid, and responsive.[39][40][41] In a head to head comparison, the CRDQ was shown to be more valid and more responsive than two other measures of dyspnoea—the Oxygen Cost Diagram and the Medical Research Council Dyspnoea Questionnaire.[41] The CRDQ has been used to assess inhaled bronchodilators,[8] theophylline,[8] and nocturnal nasal intermittent positive pressure.[42]

The St George's Respiratory Questionnaire (SGRQ) is a 76 item instrument divided into three components: symptoms, activity, and impact on daily life. This self administered questionnaire has been shown to be reproducible, valid, and responsive.[15] In a comparison with SIP, SGRQ was shown to be twice as responsive as the generic instrument. Of note, Jones and colleagues excluded questions explicitly designed to assess anxiety and depression, because other questionnaires are available for this purpose.[15]

The Oxygen Cost Diagram (OCD) represents a single vertical line with common activities listed beside it ascending in order of increasing exertional requirements. The activities range from sleeping at the bottom to brisk walking uphill at the top. Patients are asked to indicate the point above which they think their dyspnoea would limit activity. The instrument is moderately reproducible and, as already mentioned, less responsive than the CRDQ.[39]

The Baseline Dyspnoea Index (BDI) was designed by Mahler and colleagues to measure degree of dyspnoea as well as the impact of dyspnoea on an individual's life. The instrument obtains a rating from the patient on three scales: functional impairment, magnitude of task needed to evoke dyspnoea, and magnitude of effort needed to evoke dyspnoea. These are combined into a baseline score. In addition, Mahler and colleagues developed a transition dyspnoea index specifically to measure changes from the baseline condition.[3] These indices have been shown to be reproducible and valid in patients with COPD,[27][38][43] and are more responsive than the OCD.[43] Although this instrument concentrates on a single symptom of COPD, it is an important symptom and often the target of therapeutic agents. The BDI has been used to assess the value of theophylline.[7]

Features of the HRQL of patients with COPD

Description of HRQL in patients with COPD

There have been many studies describing the HRQL of patients with COPD. These studies vary in their inclusion criteria and consequently examine the HRQL of patients with varying severity of disease. The severity of disease examined has ranged from patients eligible for continuous oxygen therapy having a mean FEV_1 of 0·751 (30% of predicted)[1] to patients seen in a family practice with a mean FEV_1 of 1·86 (70% predicted).[44] Despite this heterogeneity of disease severity, a clear picture emerges showing that patients with COPD have significant decrements in their HRQL. Stewart and colleagues, using the MOS, showed that patients with COPD had decreased HRQL in all six domains of the MOS:

- physical functioning
- role functioning
- social functioning
- mental health
- health perceptions
- bodily pain.[27]

Furthermore, patients with COPD consistently scored worse on all domains than patients with hypertension, arthritis, and diabetes, and worse than those with chronic back pain on all domains except bodily pain. Similarly, McSweeny and colleagues showed that patients with severe COPD had diminished HRQL in all domains of the SIP except employment.[1] Employment is not a sensitive marker of HRQL in patients with COPD because such a large proportion of patients with COPD are retired. In the study by McSweeny *et al*, patients with COPD showed the largest decrements of HRQL in the domains of emotional disturbances (primarily depression), recreational activities, home management, and sleep and rest. Likewise, Prigatano and colleagues found wide ranging decrements of HRQL in a group of patients with COPD with moderate disease having a mean FEV_1 of 1·021.[2] It is interesting to compare the HRQL of patients from these two large studies. The patients studied by Prigatano and colleagues had a mean FEV_1 0·251 higher and a mean PaO_2 at rest 2·7 kPa (20 mm Hg) higher than those in the study by McSweeny and colleagues. Although the patients with less severe disease had

176

significantly less impairment on the physical domains of the SIP, they had very similar impairment in psychosocial domains. This suggests that, whereas degree of physical limitation is associated with severity of disease, the degree of psychosocial limitation may not be as strongly influenced by severity of disease once some threshold of COPD is reached.

An interesting feature of these studies describing the HRQL in patients with COPD is that, regardless of the instrument used or the severity of disease studied, sleep and rest are significantly disturbed.[1 2 43 37 44]

Depression, emotional dysfunction, and HRQL

A striking finding is the prominent role that depression and emotional dysfunction play in COPD. In one study patients with COPD scored lower on the mental health domain than patients with hypertension, diabetes, congestive heart failure, myocardial infarction, angina, arthritis, and chronic back pain; only patients with chronic gastrointestinal disorders scored lower in mental health.[26]

The influence of depression on the overall HRQL of a group of patients with COPD depends on its prevalence in these patients and its effect on HRQL. McSweeny and colleagues, using the MMPI, found that 42% of patients fit the category of reactive depression compared with 9% of age matched controls.[1] Light and colleagues used a questionnaire designed to detect depression (the Beck Depression Inventory—BDI) and found the same prevalence in a group of patients with less severe COPD.[38] Prigatano and colleagues used POMS to quantify depression and anxiety and found that both strongly correlated with the HRQL as measured by the SIP.[2] In fact, both anxiety and depression predicted the overall SIP score substantially better than the physiological parameters FEV_1, PaO_2, $PaCO_2$, and exercise tolerance.

Physiological measurements and HRQL

Intuitively we would expect HRQL to correlate with physiological measures of the severity of COPD. Most studies that have compared physiological measures with HRQL measures have shown correlations for the generic HRQL instruments including the SIP,[1 2 15] the QWB,[34] as well as disease specific instruments such as the BDI[3]

177

and the SGRQ.[15][16] However, not all studies show such correlations[1][36] and these correlations, when present, are not strong.

The most widely used measure of the severity of COPD is the FEV_1 which has been shown to be an accurate predictor of prognosis and survival.[45] Although most studies show that FEV_1 is statistically correlated with HRQL,[2][3][15][34][48] others have shown no significant correlation.[1][37] Even studies demonstrating a correlation have found that FEV_1 is less well correlated with HRQL than are emotional dysfunction[2][15] and dyspnoea.[15][27] Similarly, measures of oxygenation such as PaO_2 and SaO_2 are either weakly correlated with HRQL[35] or not significantly correlated.[1][2][36]

Exercise tolerance is a physiological measure which is not well predicted by ventilatory capacity or pulmonary function parameters,[46][47] but correlates with HRQL better than either FEV_1 or oxygenation correlates with HRQL.[1][2][15][34][37] Exercise tolerance also correlates with dyspnoea measures better than other parameters of pulmonary function.[3][48][49] In a study by Jones and colleagues all the correlation between pulmonary function and HRQL could be accounted for by exercise tolerance.[15]

As dyspnoea is used as a measure of HRQL, one would expect it to correlate fairly well with other HRQL instruments; in fact, dyspnoea correlates better and is a better predictor of HRQL than either pulmonary function or oxygenation.[15][27][36][44]

In general, summary statistics of correlation from different studies should be compared with caution, because studies have different entry criteria, measure different outcome measures, and use different statistical techniques. Nevertheless the squared correlation coefficients (R^2) between different variables in HRQL studies of patients with COPD have shown some homogeneity. The squared correlation coefficients of HRQL, dyspnoea and several physiological, psychological, and descriptive variables are shown in Figure 9.1. HRQL and the dyspnoea scale correlate better with one another than the physiological parameters and descriptive variables. Depression and anxiety have an intermediate correlation with HRQL and the dyspnoea scale.

In summary, several studies have shown that HRQL does correlate in the expected direction with physiological measures of COPD severity, but that the correlation is not strong or universal to all studies. These findings suggest that the physiological parameters do not predict HRQL well and that HRQL provides additional information in the assessment of patients with COPD.

178

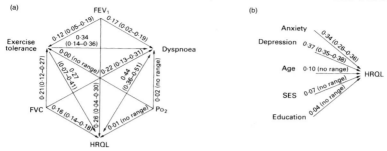

Figure 9.1   Squared correlation coefficients (R^2) of health related quality of life (HRQL), dyspnoea scale, pulmonary physiological parameters, demographic characteristics, and psychological states. The numbers represent the median of the R^2 values found with the ranges in parentheses.[1–3 15 24 34 36 38 40 48 49] R^2 can be viewed as an estimate of the proportion of the variability in HRQL or dyspnoea that is explained by a given parameter. The arrows do not imply demonstrated causality, but represent the direction of the relation of interest in understanding the role of HRQL measures. (a) Correlations of HRQL and dyspnoea with each other and with measures of pulmonary function, oxygenation, and exercise tolerance. (b) Correlations of HRQL with psychological states and demographic variables.

Comorbidity and HRQL

COPD frequently occurs in association with other diseases. Intuitively it makes sense that persons with multiple conditions would have a worse HRQL than those with just one chronic condition. Stewart and colleagues have documented the impact of comorbidity.[26] It is important to realise, however, that most clinical trials and descriptive studies of HRQL in patients with COPD have excluded significant comorbid illnesses. Consequently, the impact of comorbidity on the HRQL of patients with COPD is not well understood.

Smoking and HRQL

Another feature of HRQL is its association with continued smoking. Prigatano and colleagues found that those who continued to smoke had a significantly lower HRQL than those who had given up despite the fact that the smokers were younger and had a higher mean FEV_1.[2] Although this does not prove a causal relationship between continued smoking and HRQL, it is intriguing and worthy of further study.

179

Impact of treatment on HRQL in patients with COPD

Impact of specific treatments on HRQL in patients with COPD

Although descriptive data on the HRQL of patients with COPD are useful, the main concern of clinicians caring for patients with COPD is whether therapeutic interventions will improve HRQL. The instruments described in this review have been used to evaluate a number of specific treatments, and these studies provide insight into both specific treatments and the role of HRQL instruments in clinical research.

HRQL has been used to assess pulmonary rehabilitation and home respiratory nursing care. Ries and colleagues compared an eight week comprehensive pulmonary rehabilitation programme to an education only programme in a large, randomised trial of patients with COPD.[11] They demonstrated improved exercise capacity and symptoms with pulmonary rehabilitation, but found no difference in HRQL as measured by the SIP. Similarly, Toshima and colleagues used QWB to evaluate a comprehensive pulmonary rehabilitation programme compared with an education only control programme.[10] They demonstrated improvements in exercise tolerance with the rehabilitation programme, but showed no difference in HRQL. Bergner and colleagues showed no benefit in HRQL (using SIP and QWB) from specialised respiratory home care and concluded that current limited coverage of home care services by third party payers was appropriate.[9] Wijkstra and colleagues, however, demonstrated improved HRQL (using the CRDQ) and exercise tolerance in a randomised, controlled trial of home pulmonary rehabilitation[50] and demonstrated long term benefit in HRQL of a follow up home respiratory therapy programme.[51] It is interesting to note that the studies evaluating pulmonary rehabilitation using generic HRQL instruments have not found a benefit, whereas those using the disease specific measures have shown benefit. This may be because the generic instrument is less responsive to changes due to treatment.[18]

Guyatt and colleagues used the CRDQ to assess inhaled salbutamol and oral theophylline. In 19 patients they showed that both agents individually improved HRQL, FEV_1, exercise tolerance, and peak flow. Although some patients had additional benefit from the two agents used together, this was not statistically significant for the group.[8] Mahler and colleagues used the BDI in a crossover, double blind trial of theophylline. In this study the dyspnoea scale showed a benefit of theophylline whereas spirometry, arterial blood gases, and exercise tolerance did not significantly change.[7] More recently, McKay and colleagues have shown improved HRQL, as assessed by CRDQ, with the addition of theophylline to maximal inhaled bronchodilator therapy[52] and Kirsten and colleagues used CRDQ to demonstrate decline in HRQL after short-term withdrawal of theophylline.[53]

Van Shayck and colleagues examined the impact of routine versus symptomatic inhaled salbutamol and ipratroprium therapy on HRQL (using the NHP) and on spirometry.[37] Although they found no difference between salbutamol and ipratropium in either HRQL or spirometry, there was a significantly greater decline in FEV_1 in the group receiving continuous therapy compared with those receiving symptomatic therapy. The more rapid decline in FEV_1 was not associated with a decline in HRQL. As changes in FEV_1 and HRQL did not move in the same direction, this trial emphasises the importance of measuring HRQL rather than assuming that HRQL will change with a physiological parameter such as FEV_1.

Borson and colleagues examined the impact of antidepressant therapy on depression, HRQL (using SIP), spirometry, and exercise tolerance in 36 patients with COPD and depression.[25] They found that therapy improved not only anxiety and depression, but also HRQL. There was no significant change in FEV_1, arterial blood gases, or exercise tolerance.

The Nocturnal Oxygen Therapy Trial (NOTT) Group examined the impact of nocturnal versus continuous oxygen therapy in patients with COPD and hypoxaemia.[5] There was a decreased mortality with continuous oxygen in conjunction with a significant benefit in HRQL as assessed by the SIP (although the data were not presented). HRQL has been used to assess non-invasive positive pressure ventilation in three trials. In the Intermittent Positive Pressure Breathing (IPPB) Trial, 985 patients used either IPPB or a routine compressor nebuliser to receive inhaled bronchodilators and completed the SIP to assess HRQL.[6] The authors demonstrated no benefit of IPPB over the nebuliser in HRQL, survival, duration of hospitalisation, or lung function. In a second trial, Elliott and colleagues used the CDRQ to assess nocturnal nasal intermittent positive pressure in 12 patients, using each patient as their own historical control.[42] They found improved sleep time and sleep efficiency, but no change in HRQL. Finally, Jones and colleagues recently examined nocturnal nasal pressure support ventilation plus long term oxygen therapy compared with oxygen therapy alone in a small, but well designed, randomised trial of patients with stable hypercapnic respiratory failure due to COPD.[54] They found significant improvements in HRQL as well as daytime arterial Pao_2 and $Paco_2$ with the nocturnal nasal positive pressure ventilation.

Overview of HRQL in therapeutic trials for patients with COPD

These trials show a range of possible outcomes from using HRQL instruments. The HRQL instrument may agree with other outcome measures and thereby provide additional evidence either for or against the use of a specific treatment. The instrument may show no benefit when other outcomes such as survival show clear benefit. In this case it is important that clinicians and patients be aware of this discrepancy and consider it in the decision to use the treatment. If the benefit of treatment is considered to outweigh the lack of improvement in HRQL, the patient's awareness of this lack of benefit in HRQL may minimise disappointment with the treatment and consequent non-compliance. Finally, HRQL instruments may show a benefit when traditional outcomes do not, and these instruments may allow patients to receive important and effective treatment that would otherwise be assessed as ineffective.

Applicability of HRQL measures to clinical practice

Use of HRQL measures in clinical practice

In general the practising clinician assesses the HRQL of a patient with COPD by taking a careful history, eliciting symptoms, and assessing how these symptoms affect functional capacity and ability to perform the recreational and social activities that the patient enjoys. The practising clinician generally does not need an HRQL instrument to perform this assessment. There may, however, be circumstances in which these instruments may be directly useful to the practising clinician as a self-administered generic or disease specific HRQL instrument for patients to complete in the waiting room. This practice may identify specific areas of concern or changes over time that might not become obvious during routine visits. For this purpose the HRQL instrument would need to be not only reproducible, valid, and responsive, but also easily administered and interpreted in the clinical setting. Candidate instruments would include the MOS[56][57] and the SGRQ.

In addition, an HRQL instrument could be useful in the N of 1 trial. Guyatt and colleagues have described the utility and practice of N of 1 randomised controlled trials in detail and this technique can be very useful in assessing an individual's response to different therapeutic approaches. In the N of 1 trial, HRQL is an ideal outcome measure as the point of these trials is usually to determine the treatment which provides patients with the best HRQL.[17][58]

Lessons to the clinician regarding HRQL in COPD

Previous research has pointed out several important, but not widely known, features of the HRQL of patients with COPD. First, maximal improvement in physiological measures of disease severity such as FEV_1 or oxygenation may not be sufficient for maximal improvement of HRQL. If we are interested in improving HRQL we must assess it directly. As a corollary of this point, it is possible to improve HRQL without changing any physiological measures of disease severity. The use of antidepressants in individuals with COPD and depression improved HRQL without changing FEV_1 or exercise tolerance.[27]

A second important lesson to the clinician provided by the studies of HRQL is that COPD has a major impact on specific facets of HRQL that might not be obvious, including depression, anxiety, sleep, and rest. It is not clear whether depression and anxiety cause a decrease in HRQL or vice versa. It seems likely that there is a complex interdependence of these factors, but it is clear that treating depression and anxiety can improve HRQL.[27]

A final generic lesson of these studies is that individuals vary as to what they consider to be the most important aspects of HRQL and these are not well correlated with disease severity, exercise tolerance, or other terms familiar to clinicians. In the assessment of an individual patient's HRQL it is important to ask directly what each person values about his or her life, including religious beliefs, value system, and his or her priorities. This is especially important in COPD because the disease predisposes patients to acute respiratory failure, where it is often appropriate to consider withholding or withdrawing life support measures such as mechanical ventilation. This decision depends on the likelihood of a reversible component and on the patient's acceptance or rejection of the treatment based on risks and benefits offered. The patient's response may depend on their HRQL before the acute event. Often patients will be unable to make a decision about life support based on a hypothetical scenario before the acute event, but early discussion will give clinicians and family members a better understanding of the patient's views should he or she be unable to participate once in respiratory failure. Without these discussions many physicians and families do not have a good understanding of the patient's wishes. This was documented by Uhlmann and colleagues who asked patients, their spouses, and physicians whether they wished cardiopulmonary resuscitation and mechanical ventilation to be given to the patient if he or she became critically ill. In about 40% of cases the wishes of both the patient's spouse and the physician differed from those of the patient.[59]

Summary

Assessment of HRQL is an important feature of the care of patients with chronic disease. The instruments will be used increasingly to assess the quality of life of patients with specific diseases and to help assess the impact of treatment. In addition, as outcome assessment becomes an increasing part of health care technology, HRQL will become a common outcome measure. To assess the value of an HRQL measure clinicians must have a basic understanding of the field of HRQL assessment. Clinicians should expect the instrument used to be reproducible, valid, and responsive in patients with the disease under study. Studies describing new HRQL instruments should be expected to show the need for, or advantage of, a new instrument as opposed to one already developed and tested.

HRQL instruments have provided important insights into the lives of patients with moderate to severe COPD. They have also been essential in indicating that some treatments improve the lives of patients with COPD whereas others do not. We can expect that the HRQL instruments will continue this role in future research.

Acknowledgment

Supported in part by the Robert Wood Johnson Foundation and the Health Services Research and Development Field Program, Seattle Veterans Affairs Medical Center. Dr Curtis is a Robert Wood Johnson

Clinical Scholar. The views expressed herein are those of the authors and are not necessarily the views of the Robert Wood Johnson Foundation.

1 McSweeny AJ, Grant I, Heaton RK, Adams KM, Timms RM. Life quality of patients with chronic obstructive pulmonary disease. *Arch Intern Med* 1982;**142**: 473–8.
2 Prigatano GP, Wright EC, Levin D. Quality of life and its predictors in patients with mild hypoxemia and chronic obstructive pulmonary disease. *Arch Intern Med* 1984;**144**:1613–9.
3 Mahler D, Weinber D, Wells C, Feinstein A. The measurement of dyspnea: contents, interobserver agreement, and physiologic correlates of two new clinical indexes. *Chest* 1984;**85**:751–8.
4 Guyatt G, Townsend M, Berman L, Pugsley S. Quality of life in patients with chronic airflow limitation. *Br J Dis Chest* 1987;**81**:45–54.
5 Nocturnal Oxygen Therapy Trial Group. Continuous or nocturnal oxygen therapy in hypoxemic chronic obstructive lung disease. *Ann Intern Med* 1980; **93**:391–8.
6 Intermittent Positive Pressure Breathing Trial Group. Intermittent positive pressure breathing therapy of chronic obstructive pulmonary disease. *Ann Intern Med* 1983;**99**:612–20.
7 Mahler DA, Matthay RA, Snyder PE, Wells CK, Loke J. Sustained-release theophylline reduces dyspnea in nonreversible obstructive airway disease. *Am Rev Respir Dis* 1985;**131**:22–5.
8 Guyatt GH, Townsend M, Pugsley SO, *et al.* Bronchodilators in chronic airflow limitation: effects on airway function, exercise capacity, and quality of life. *Am Rev Respir Dis* 1987;**135**:1069–74.
9 Bergner M, Hudson LD, Conrad DA, *et al.* The cost and efficacy of home care for patients with chronic lung disease. *Med Care* 1988;**26**:566–79.
10 Toshima MT, Kaplan RM, Ries AL. Experimental evaluation of rehabilitation in chronic obstructive pulmonary disease: short-term effects on exercise endurance and health status. *Health Psychol* 1990;**9**:237–52.
11 Ries AL, Kaplan RM, Limberg TM, Prewitt LM. Effects of pulmonary rehabilitation on physiologic and psychosocial outcomes in patients with chronic obstructive pulmonary disease. *Ann Intern Med* 1995;**122**:823–32.
12 Kirshner B, Guyatt G. A methodological framework for assessing health indices. *J Chronic Dis* 1985;**38**:27–36.
13 Deyo R. Measuring the functional status of patients with low back pain. *Arch Phys Med Rehabil* 1988;**69**:1044–53.
14 Feinstein AR. Clinical biostatistics: hard science, soft data, and the challenges of choosing clinical variables in research. *Clin Pharmacol Ther* 1977;**22**:485–98.
15 Jones P, Quirk FH, Baveystock CM, Littlejohns P. A self-complete measure of health status for chronic airflow limitation. The St George's Respiratory Questionnaire. *Am Rev Respir Dis* 1992;**145**:1321–7.
16 Wijkstra PJ, Ten Vergert EM, van der Mark TW, *et al.* Relation of lung function, maximal inspiratory pressure, dyspnoea, and quality of life with exercise capacity in patients with chronic obstructive pulmonary disease. *Thorax* 1994;**49**:468–72.
17 Guyatt GG, Feeny D, Patrick D. Issues in quality-of-life measurement in clinical trials. *Controlled Clin Trials* 1991;**12**:81S–90S.
18 Jones PW. Issues concerning health-related quality of life in COPD. *Chest* 1995; **5**(suppl):187–93.
19 Mills JL. Data torturing. *N Engl J Med* 1993;**329**:1196–9.
20 Jaeschke R, Guyatt GH, Keller J, Singer J. Interpreting changes in quality-of-life score in N of 1 randomized trials. *Controlled Clin Trials* 1991;**12**:226S–33S.

21 Pocock SJ. A perspective on the role of quality-of-life assessment in clinical trials. *Controlled Clin Trials* 1991;**12**:257S–65S.
22 Bergner M, Bobbitt RA, Carter WB, Gilson BS. The sickness impact profile: development and final revision of a health status measure. *Med Care* 1981;**19**: 787–805.
23 McSweeny AJ, Heaton RK, Grant I, Cugell D, Solliday N, Timms R. Chronic obstructive pulmonary disease; socioemotional adjustment and life quality. *Chest* 1980;**77**:309–11.
24 Jones P, Baveystock CM, Littlejohns P. Relationships between general health measured with the sickness impact profile and respiratory symptoms, physiological measures, and mood in patients with chronic airflow limitation. *Am Rev Respir Dis* 1989;**140**:1538–43.
25 Borson S, McDonald GJ, Gayle T, Deffebach M, Lakshminarayan S, Van Tuinen C. Improvement in mood, physical symptoms, and function with nortriptyline for depression in patients with chronic obstructive pulmonary disease. *Psychosomatics* 1992;**33**:190–201.
26 Stewart AL, Greenfield S, Hays RD, *et al.* Functional status and well-being of patients with chronic conditions: results from the medical outcomes study. *JAMA* 1989;**262**:907–13.
27 Mahler DA, Faryniarz K, Tomlinsom D, *et al.* Impact of dyspnea and physiologic function on general health status in patients with chronic obstructive pulmonary disease. *Chest* 1992;**102**:395–401.
28 Ware JE, Sherbourne CD. The MOS 36-item short form health survey (SF-36). *Med Care* 1992;**30**:473–83.
29 McHorney CA, Ware JE, Rogers W, Raczek AE, Lu J. The validity and relative precision of MOS short- and long-form health status scales and Dartmouth COOP charts. *Med Care* 1992;**30**:MS253–65.
30 Mahler DA, Mackowiak JI. Evaluation of the Short-Form 36-Item questionnaire to measure health-related quality of life in patients with COPD. *Chest* 1995; **107**:1585–9.
31 Fanshel S, Bush JW. A health-status index and its application to health-services outcomes. *Operations Res* 1970;**18**:1021–66.
32 Kaplan RM, Bush JW, Berry CC. Category rating versus magnitude estimation for measuring levels of well-being. *Med Care* 1979;**17**:501–21.
33 Anderson JP, Kaplan RM, Berry CC, Bush JW, Rumbaut RG. Interday reliability of function assessment for a health status measure: the quality of well-being scale. *Med Care* 1989;**27**:1076–83.
34 Kaplan RM, Atkins CJ, Timms R. Validity of a quality of well-being scale as an outcome measure in chronic obstructive pulmonary disease. *J Chronic Dis* 1984;**37**:85–95.
35 Hunt SM, McKenna SP, McEwen J, Backett EM, Williams J, Papp E. A quantitative approach to perceived health status: a validation study. *J Epidemiol Community Health* 1980;**34**:281–6.
36 Alonso J, Anto JM, Gonzalez M, Fiz JA, Izquierdo J, Morera J. Measurement of general health status of non-oxygen-dependent chronic obstructive pulmonary disease patients. *Med Care* 1992;**30**:MS125–35.
37 van Shayck CP, Rutten-van Molken MPMH, van Doorslaer EKA, Folgering H, van Weel C. Two-year bronchodilator treatment in patients with mild airflow obstruction: contradictory effects on lung function and quality of life. *Chest* 1992;**102**:1384–91.
38 Light RW, Merrill EJ, Despars JA, Gordon GH, Mutalipassi LR. Prevalence of depression and anxiety in patients with COPD: relationship to functional capacity. *Chest* 1985;**87**:35–8.
39 Guyatt G, Berman L, Townsend M, Pugsley S, Chambers L. A measure of quality of life for clinical trials in chronic lung disease. *Thorax* 1987;**42**:773–8.

40 Guyatt G, Townsend M, Keller J, Singer J, Nogradi S. Measuring functional status in chronic lung disease: conclusions from a randomized control trial. *J Respir Med* 1989;**83**:293–7.

41 Wijkstra PJ, TenVergert EN, Van Altena RV, *et al.* Reliability and validity of the chronic respiratory questionnaire (CRDQ). *Thorax* 1994;**49**:465–7.

42 Elliott MW, Simonds AK, Carroll MP, Wedzicha JA, Branthwaite MA. Domiciliary nocturnal nasal intermittent positive pressure ventilation in hypercapnic respiratory failure due to chronic obstructive lung disease: effects on sleep and quality of life. *Thorax* 1992;**47**:342–8.

43 Mahler D, Rosiello R, Harver A, Lentine T, McGovern J, Daubenspeck J. Comparison of clinical dyspnea ratings and psychophysical measurements of respiratory sensation in obstructive airway disease. *Am Rev Respir Dis* 1987; **135**:1229–33.

44 Schrier A, Dekker FW, Kaptein AA, Dijkman JH. Quality of life in elderly patients with chronic nonspecific lung disease seen in family practice. *Chest* 1990;**98**:894–9.

45 Hudson LD. Survival data in patients with acute and chronic lung disease. *Am Rev Respir Dis* 1990;**140**:519–24.

46 Killian KL, LeBlanc P, Martin DH, Summers E, Jones NL, Campbell EJM. Exercise capacity and ventilatory, circulatory, and symptom limitation in patients with chronic airflow limitation. *Am Rev Respir Dis* 1992;**146**:935–40.

47 Morgan AD, Peck DF, Buchanan DR, McHardy GJR. Effect of attitudes and beliefs on exercise tolerance in chronic bronchitis. *BMJ* 1983;**286**:171–3.

48 McGavin C, Artvinli M, Naoe H, McHardly G. Dyspnoea, disability, and distance walked: comparison of estimates of exercise performance in respiratory disease. *BMJ* 1978;**2**:241–3.

49 Guyatt G, Thompson P, Berman L, *et al.* How should we measure function in patients with chronic heart and lung disease. *J Chronic Dis* 1985;**38**:517–24.

50 Wijkstra PJ, Van Altena RV, Kraan J, Otten V, Postma DS, Koeter GH. Quality of life in patients with chronic obstructive pulmonary disease after rehabilitation at home. *Eur Respir J* 1994;**7**:269–73.

51 Wijkstra PJ, TenVergert EM, van Altena R, *et al.* Long term benefits of rehabilitation at home on quality of life and exercise tolerance in patients with chronic obstructive pulmonary disease. *Thorax* 1995;**50**:824–8.

52 McKay SE, Howie CA, Thomson AH, Whiting B, Addis GJ. Value of theophylline treatment in patients handicapped by chronic obstructive lung disease. *Thorax* 1993;**48**:227–32.

53 Kirsten DK, Wegner RE, Jorres RA, Magnussen H. Effects of theophylline withdrawal in severe chronic obstructive pulmonary disease. *Chest* 1993;**104**: 1101–7.

54 Jones DJM, Paul EA, Jones PW, Wedzicha JA. Nasal pressure support ventilation plus oxygen compared with oxygen therapy alone in hypercapnic COPD. *Am J Respir Crit Care Med* 1995;**152**:538–44.

55 Rubenstein LV, Calkins DR, Young RT, *et al.* Improving patient function: a randomized trial of functional disability screening. *Ann Intern Med* 1989;**111**: 836–42.

56 Calkins DR, Rubenstein LV, Cleary PD, *et al.* Failure of physicians to recognize functional disability in ambulatory patients. *Ann Intern Med* 1991;**114**:451–4.

57 Guyatt GH, Keller JL, Jaeschke R, Rosenbloom D, Adachi JD, Newhouse MT. The n-of-1 randomized controlled trial: clinical usefulness. *Ann Intern Med* 1990;**112**:293–9.

58 Uhlmann RF, Pearlman RA, Cain K. Physicians' and spouses' predictions of elderly patients' resuscitation preferences. *J Gerontol* 1988;**43**:M115–M21.

10 Setting up a pulmonary rehabilitation programme

CJ CLARK

The content of pulmonary rehabilitation schemes varies considerably among centres. This is likely to remain the case until detailed research has shown which components are most valuable. The emphasis on outpatient, inpatient, and home-based programmes also differs widely. In this chapter a stepwise approach to setting up a pulmonary rehabilitation programme is described. It is recognised, however, that schemes need to meet local needs, and that a variety of approaches may be equally successful.

Identifications of aims

The programme's rationale is to maximise the functions of daily living for individual patients with chronic disabling lung disease by introducing a comprehensive process of assessment and treatment. The focus will be on chronic obstructive pulmonary disease as the predominant chronic lung disease to consider first, and then other applications of pulmonary rehabilitation will be mentioned briefly.

Implicit in the approach of this chapter is the assumption that routine services in the United Kingdom and other countries already contain many components which address patients' needs and do not require duplication. The objective in setting up pulmonary rehabilitation is therefore to *complement* rather than *replace* existing services. The advantage of this approach is that it is:

1 Less financially prohibitive to add to existing resources
2 More likely to result in an efficient use of the resources specifically required for pulmonary rehabilitation

3 The process of reviewing current practice is likely to identify deficits and thereby improve the standards of routine care.

The following are the possible components of pulmonary rehabilitation that may include those aspects of patient care not currently part of routine service and thus could be incorporated into a programme:[1]

- Pharmacological therapy
- Education
- Physical therapy
- Exercise conditioning
- Occupational therapy
- Psychosocial support
- Follow up treatment
- Oxygen therapy
- Nutritional therapy
- Respiratory muscles.

District general hospital chest clinics usually provide for prescription of drug therapy, demonstration of inhaler technique, basic explanation of the disease process, and referral for traditional physiotherapy breathing techniques, and deal with special requirements such as long term oxygen treatment (LTOT) or home ventilator therapy. Thus some components of pulmonary rehabilitation are "already in progress". On the other hand, investigation of activities of daily living, psychosocial function, nutritional status and, in particular, exercise prescription can be viewed as essential prerequisites for successful comprehensive pulmonary rehabilitation, and it is therefore important to concentrate on these aspects of care if not routinely available.

Deciding the infrastructure requirements

Staff requirements

Programme director

A chest physician should undertake this role which includes medicolegal responsibility for patient care during rehabilitation. He or she should be responsible for:

1 Aspects of programme design
2 Accurate assessment of suitability of patients for inclusion

189

3 Ensuring full and informed written consent by the patient
4 Appropriate programme prescription for the individual patient
5 Quality control of programme administration by staff
6 Ensuring continuity of care between the programme and general practice.

In addition to these administrative responsibilities it is important to leave time to be practically involved in the training programme. This will ensure both that enthusiasm is allowed to develop and that the programme is viewed by the administration as a routine rather than optional service. In practice this requires one fixed session for a pulmonary rehabilitation medical assessment clinic plus time availability to see patients on an ad hoc basis. This last commitment is unlikely to be frequent if the programme is well structured with supportive staff.

Assistant medical staff

Ideally two to three sessional commitments per week of middle grade medical staff should be allocated to the pulmonary rehabilitation programme. One session is for the medical assessment clinic. This should be a fixed commitment, and should be recognised as contributing to the doctor's postgraduate training programme. The second session is required for medical supervision of exercise testing (this may already be covered within existing pulmonary investigation facilities). A third ongoing commitment is valuable for dealing on an ad hoc basis with patient problems arising during rehabilitation. This can be viewed as an extension of the usual resident staff commitment to daily in-hospital referral of patients with chest problems.

Physiotherapist (see chapter 6)

Pulmonary rehabilitation provides an exciting new opportunity for physiotherapy, extending from the traditional role in lung disease management to a central role in conducting exercise sessions—a core activity in pulmonary rehabilitation. The techniques of breathing re-training are well established adjuncts to the management of chronic disabling breathlessness and routine physiotherapy services normally include a provision for treatment of selected patients. Applied exercise physiology is generally less comprehensively covered in physiotherapy training although important in the context of this widening role. Assume, therefore,

190

that some additional in-service staff training will be required before formally commencing pulmonary rehabilitation.

The following are recommended for physiotherapist in-service training:

1 The principles of individualised exercise prescription[2] should be studied.
2 The local leisure centre fitness programmes for normal individuals should be visited to obtain some experience of standard components used. Advice, particularly concerning "start up" programmes for previously sedentary individuals, should be taken. Commercial organisations are consumer responsive and aspects such as gymnasium lighting and decor, together with careful choice of music, are essential considerations. Patients are also consumers and compliance is enhanced in circumstances that are bright and cheerful (the programme should appear less work and more a "leisure" pursuit).
3 The basic physiology of exercise limitation in lung disease[4 5] should be covered through seminars arranged by the programme director.

Calculation of physiotherapy sessional commitments requires an estimation of the likely patient throughput. For example:

No. patients per session	8–10 maximum
Sessions per week per patient group	2 hospital (plus 1 unsupervised)
Duration of patient programme	3 months
No. physiotherapy exercise sessions weekly:	
aerobic/mobility	5
multigym	2
conditioning	2
programme for the "severe" patient	1
Physiotherapy assessment clinic	1 session/week

The minimal physiotherapy commitment likely for pulmonary rehabilitation of 30 patients over three months with an annual turnover of 120 patients would be six sessions—that is, 24 hours/week.

191

Training in techniques for aiding expectoration and breathing re-training should not be devolved from the routine service to pulmonary rehabilitation as "start-up" funding should be allocated to new and not to existing services.

Occupational therapy

This an essential requirement to ensure that adequate time and expertise are available to identify problems—that is, those activities of daily living that can be improved. This would require one session/week (clinic or occupational therapy departmental assessment) and an optional session/week for home visits on an ad hoc basis.

Nurse liaison

The process of pulmonary rehabilitation involves not only the hospital programmes but also liaison with primary care workers. The role of a nurse will be to conduct a weekly clinic whose function is:

1 Coordinating between the referral clinic, the pulmonary rehabilitation programme, and between the various programme assessments
2 To conduct patient questionnaire assessments of quality of life and psychosocial functioning at the outset and on completion of the programme
3 Educational, to improve the patient's understanding of his or her illness (the information to be discussed is summarised in the box)
4 Before programme completion to ensure that adequate follow up programmes for self management are established with written guidelines and instructions for primary care professionals (general practitioners, practice nurses)
5 Collation of nutritional assessment and advice from the dietician, including documentation and communication with the general practitioner
6 Additional home assessment of selected patients, usually those with severe disease where required.

The programme should allow for four nurse liaison sessions/week (one assessment clinic, one administration/coordination session, one educational group session, and one "floating" session for home and health centre liaison visits). Note that such visits require a budget for mileage allowance.

Educational topics for discussion

Normal anatomy and physiology of the lungs and heart

Types of lung disease and other conditions that affect the function of the lungs

Abnormal anatomy and physiology associated with pulmonary disorders

Types of medical tests that will be performed, procedures for testing, and interpretation and significance of the results

Medications: drug actions, description of products, desired beneficial effects, side effects, techniques of self administration, and methods to assist patients to remember to take the medication

Breathing exercises, including whether to perform them at rest, during exercise, or during recovery from exercise or stress

Energy conservation techniques associated with activities of daily living

Relaxation techniques and methods to reduce stress

Emotional aspects of chronic disease

Nutrition and fluid intake

Causes of shortness of breath

Role of exercise and physical fitness

Recognising problems associated with their disease: infection, hypercapnia, hypoxia

How to treat symptoms

Who to call for problems

From Gilmartin.[3]

Facilities required for initial and ongoing patient assessment

The programme can be conducted as an additional outpatient service in which all assessments take place within existing clinic facilities. A total commitment of three half day sessions should be allowed at the outset—that is, one medical, one nursing, and one physiotherapy/occupational therapy. The appointments should be grouped by patient category to ensure efficient use of time in dealing with issues relevant to that particular group. The different role of each session will be described below. It is, however, useful at this stage to consider the process of pulmonary rehabilitation as in some ways analogous to modern management of diabetes where outpatient services divide assessment and management among doctor, nurse, and paramedical staff under overall medical supervision. Similarly, not every patient needs to be processed through every aspect of pulmonary rehabilitation providing that the referral process has included an accurate assessment of needs.

Medical assessment

Apart from the initial and final medical visits, each patient will require an assessment after six weeks on the programme to record clinical progress and to decide whether he or she remains fit to continue. Progress reports from the physiotherapist and nurse coordinator should be available at this visit which can be short and focused on pulmonary rehabilitation as routine patient care remains primarily the responsibility of the general practitioner. This clinic also allows the nurse and/or physiotherapist access for extra medical assessments if required during pulmonary rehabilitation, in addition to the routine visits.

Nursing assessment

Each patient completes the functional questionnaires at the first visit (before the nurse appointment if a self administered questionnaire is used) and the findings are discussed. The patient's understanding of his or her illness is then explored using guidelines given in the box, and finally the programme's objectives are outlined.

Generic and disease specific quality of life questionnaires have been reviewed in chapter 9. All of our patients have a disease specific quality of life assessment combined with a short validated questionnaire for psychological function,[6] and patients with moderate to severe impairment also have an assessment of activities of daily living.[7] A single page of "self efficacy" questionnaire[8] is also helpful to determine whether the patient feels able to comply with the programme. It is then possible to set realistic targets for improvement in those areas identified as deficient in the questionnaires by agreement between the nurse and patient. This must be recorded in brief on a patient proforma which also contains pre-prepared information about his or her illness and the programme content. The topics discussed and the outcome of the interview should also be recorded in a pulmonary rehabilitation case sheet which is used for all aspects of the programme.

Paramedical (physiotherapist/occupational therapist) assessment

Although many of the issues that the physiotherapist requires to discuss with the patient are covered during evaluation, it is useful to include this session in planning to arrange group meetings and more detailed discussion where appropriate. Important topics include basic principles behind training, dealing with simple problems which occur such as muscle discomfort after exercise, planning increased activity, and methods of continuing involvement in exercise on completion of the programme. These aspects are covered in detail in chapter 6.

The occupational therapist's involvement in a fixed weekly session is a valuable commitment and the decision to arrange occupational therapy assessment should be made if the initial evaluation of the patient's illness severity and functional handicap by the programme nurse using the activities of daily living questionnaire reveals a need for practical assistance with activities of daily living. Occupational therapy services may already have been provided by the general practitioner or be available from that source, in which case the results of a single pulmonary rehabilitation assessment can be communicated to the community occupational therapist for implementation.

Additional support services

Clinical psychology—Liaison with the clinical psychology services is helpful at the outset to explain the programme objectives and to set up a referral process so that patients found on routine screening to have psychological problems can be seen and treated expeditiously as part of the pulmonary rehabilitation programme. Expert advice can also be obtained regarding the interpretation of the psychological questionnaire and indications for patient referral for further assessment. Our policy jointly agreed with clinical psychology is to use the nurse screening process following set criteria obtained from the questionnaire to determine referral requirements.

Dietetics—The dietetics department also requires to be informed of the specific requirements of the programme and given written information about the current role of nutritional assessment in the management of chronic obstructive pulmonary disease.[9 10]

Facilities required for evaluation of lung and exercise function

Although specialist units have the full range of lung and exercise testing facilities, this chapter concentrates on pulmonary rehabilitation within district general hospitals with more basic lung function laboratories. Usual facilities will range from dynamic spirometric testing alone to measurement of lung volumes and diffusing capacity (TLCO). Simple spirometric testing is required for pulmonary rehabilitation to provide some measurement of disease severity which is unlikely to alter as a consequence of pulmonary rehabilitation.[11] Although TLCO is a useful indicator of resting gas exchange it is not essential, but measurements of arterial blood gas tensions at rest and oxygen saturation during exercise will be required to determine oxygen requirements during pulmonary rehabilitation. All patients should be screened during exercise and not just those considered to be "at risk" (resting hypoxaemia, known history of desaturation, low TLCO).

Where units do not have facilities for progressive incremental exercise testing incorporating gas exchange measurements, adequate exercise evaluation for pulmonary rehabilitation can be performed using "field" tests (six and 12 minute walk tests, shuttle test[12 13]) or just a treadmill test using the Bruce protocol[14] to evaluate overall (whole body) exercise capacity.

As most pulmonary rehabilitation programmes involve submaximal endurance training, it is also helpful to measure endurance time and work during submaximal exercise on a treadmill before and after pulmonary rehabilitation.

Finally, for programmes concentrating on individual muscle group training (conditioning and multigym), additional exercise testing is performed in the gymnasium by the physiotherapist. This consists of measuring the effects of training on the endurance of specific muscle exercise repetitions before and after pulmonary rehabilitation.

Patients with known or suspected ischaemic heart disease should be excluded from pulmonary rehabilitation exercise programmes because the additional risk of adverse events is high. All patients should have a 12 lead ECG performed during initial evaluation and immediately after maximal exercise testing as a medicolegal precaution to identify ischaemic heart disease.

Exercise protocols

Walking tests—These field tests measure maximal exercise tolerance (distance walked). Provided that conditions are standardised—for example, repeated in the same corridor with the same supervisor—they provide a convenient, valid method of longitudinal assessment in individual patients. Familiarisation with the test is essental before the formal test.

Treadmill tests—The work rate increments in the Bruce protocol are given in Figure 10.1. It allows for limited tolerance in patients

196

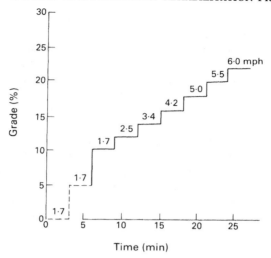

Figure 10.1   Work rate increments in the Bruce protocol.[14]

with ischaemic heart disease by reducing the increments of work rate compared with protocols for normal healthy individuals, and is therefore suitable for patients with lung disease. The graded work increments are "enforced" and the test is more reproducible than walk tests. After familiarisation a single test is usually reliable and adequate before pulmonary rehabilitation.

Treadmill endurance time and work are obtained from steady state exercise at a predetermined submaximal work rate. Although previous estimation of maximal exercise on the treadmill is useful in deciding the approximate treadmill incline and speed required (usually the increments that produce a heart rate of 70% of "symptom limited" maximum heart rate), it is not essential. Familiarity with the performance of endurance tests often allows a "best guess" at the most appropriate increments to use for individual patients. The author uses the "rule of 5's" assessment,[15] however, to give an indication of maximal tolerable work increments for exercise endurance in individual patients and this has several advantages:

1 It is simple to apply, requiring only a treadmill, heart rate monitor, and evaluation of the patients' symptoms
2 It can be used to measure endurance time—that is, if a tolerable work rate is identified the assessment can be continued to exhaustion

3 The information can be used by the physiotherapist to predict the impact of breathlessness during performance of endurance training and to decide on the best programme for the patient.

Measurement of endurance at the relatively high work rates involved also ensures that testing time is not too demanding—that is, inordinately long. Prior familiarisation with the treadmill is advisable because sustained patient motivation is required with endurance tests to ensure a valid end point.[16]

Total endurance work (joules) performed is given by the formula:[16]

Power (W) $[0.536 \times wt$ (kg) $\times 0.625 \times speed$ (kph) $\times 0.1635] \times time$ in s

Note that in this equation work is underestimated because incline cannot be taken into account, but this is not a problem as incline is unchanged in evaluation of the patient's endurance before and after pulmonary rehabilitation.

All of these tests provide target end points which can be used as indicators of improved exercise tolerance, the magnitude of which will vary between patients depending on a number of factors including the extent of disability on commencement, and the degree to which the patient complies with the programme.

Facilities required for exercise programmes

There are two distinct modes of exercise programme requiring separate facilities:

1 Aerobic/mobility training
2 Multigym "weight" training.

Both can be supplemented by instruction to patients to incorporate simple walking into their daily routine. This requires planning—that is, tolerable distances and areas to walk need to be identified by the patient and a log kept of progress in order to document fully the exercise being undertaken during pulmonary rehabilitation.

Although programmes for aerobic/mobility training may vary, they require adequate floor space and heating as provided in a typical indoor gymnasium. Unike aerobics classes in healthy adults, however, the instructor not only supervises the group but also monitors each individual patient. The size of group at any session is therefore limited to 8–10 patients, and the overall gym area need not be large ($225 \, m^2$ is adequate).

Multigym training uses specialised equipment to provide a "circuit" of exercises for individual muscle groups. A separate exercise area is essential and again this need not be large as there are the same constraints on patient numbers as already described. Each item of equipment may stand alone, but a combined multiuser apparatus containing up to eight items with one or two extra stand alone items to complete the requirements provides for efficient use of limited space. The box lists the range of equipment items which have been incorporated in the multigym, together with the muscle groups they are designed to condition. A similar approach has recently improved endurance in patients with COPD.[16] Note that cardiopulmonary resuscitation facilities with staff training are essential for all exercise programmes.

Implementing exercise rehabilitation programmes

Training benefits are usually seen by six weeks[2 16] and this may suffice if a high patient throughput is essential, but in our experience a 12 week programme is preferable. The longer time often provides a depth of experience about the relationship between exercise and the individual's disease which can be of permanent benefit after the programme has finished.

Suggested endurance training for patients with mild COPD

For endurance training to achieve measurable improvements in fitness the following variables need to be controlled:[17]

1 Frequency of exercise should be a minimum of three times weekly
2 Duration per session should be a minimum of 20 minutes
3 Exercise intensity per session should not be less than two thirds maximum work rate achievable if the patient had no lung disease
4 A programme timescale not less than six weeks should be used.

This is a group programme conducted in two sessions weekly in the hospital gymnasium supplemented by an unsupervised home session. Patients can join and leave the programme on an ad hoc basis because within a set session the patient performs his or her own exercise prescription. At the first session an exercise programme suitable for sedentary individuals commencing training for the first time is given, and the target intensity is that producing a heart rate

Multigym exercises designed to improve skeletal muscle strength and endurance

These exercises do not require to be performed in a set order. They must, however, be preceded by a five minute period of warm up exercises prescribed by the physiotherapist. Weight ranges are given for each item of equipment

Supine bench press
Exercises the chest, front of shoulders, and rear upper arm. Position: the patient lies with shoulders below the handlebar and presses upwards until elbows locked then returns to resting position. Ten repetitions continuously over approximately 20 seconds. The breathing pattern should coincide with repetitions. Rest between sets until Borg score is less than 3. Weight range 12–74 kg with 2 kg increments to 22 kg, 4 kg increments thereafter

Power squat
Exercises the buttocks, thighs and low back. Position: the patient stands facing the weights, squats down beneath shoulder pads and grasps bar. Pushes up until knees lock straight then carefully returns to resting position. Repetitions, breathing pattern, and rest periods as for previous exercise. Weight range 20–90 kg with 5 kg increments

Calf raise
Exercises the ankle extensors. Position: at same equipment station as previous exercise, stand with shoulders beneath the pads and knees straight and locked, feet flat. Lift heels raising weights until fully extended on tip of toes only. Repetitions as for first exercise. Weight range 20–90 kg with 5 kg increments

Latissimus pull down
Exercises the large back muscles, upper chest and front upper arms. Position: stand facing weights, grasp overhead bar and pull down to midchest and return carefully to resting position. Repetitions as for first exercise. Weight range 0–70 kg with 5 kg increments

Upright rowing
Exercises the shoulder muscles and elbow flexors. Position: stand facing the low pulley, draw weight to thighs then lift handlebar from thighs to shoulder height returning carefully to thighs. Repetitions as for first exercise. Weight range 5–65 kg with increments of 2·5 kg to 15 kg then 5 kg increments

---

Multigym exercises designed to improve skeletal muscle strength and endurance—*continued*

Leg press

Exercises all lower limb muscles in coordination fashion. Position: sitting with knees bent and feet on rotating foot plate, push till knees fully extended leading with heels, not toes and return carefully to resting position. Repetitions as for first exercise but allow 30 seconds for each set. Weight range 32–208 kg with 11 kg increments

Leg extension

Exercises the quadriceps. Position: sit with back to weights and feet hooked under lower pads. Extend at knees until fully locked and return carefully to resting position. Repetitions etc as for previous exercise. Weight range 7–61 kg with 3 kg increments

Leg curls

Exercises the hamstrings. Position: lie flat on bench face down with heels under padded roller. Curl legs till heels are directly above knees then carefully return to resting position. Repetitions as for leg press. Weight range 7–61 kg with 3 kg increments

Allow up to 30 minutes for completion of the programme inclusive of warm up, rest periods between sets and different stations plus warm down at end of session

---

of about 70% of predicted maximum. Heart rate is variably increased in some patients with chronic obstructive pulmonary disease[18] and can only be used as an approximate expression of work intensity. If the patient is limited by breathlessness the physiotherapist modifies the programme to the maximal exercise intensity tolerable, and the wrist heart rate monitor is then used to help reproduce the same intensity in subsequent sessions by controlling the frequency of exercise repetitions, whereas the programme content is standardised in all other respects. Though breathlessness may require modification for individual subjects, significant improvements in exercise tolerance can still be achieved.[19] Patients who complete the programme without modification can be anticipated to improve exercise capacity ($\dot{V}o_2$max) by the same amount as normal sedentary subjects—that is, up to 30%.[17]

Multigym weight training for patients with moderate disease

The principle involved in training specific muscle groups is repetition of "isotonic" contractions—that is, against a fixed weight, usually 60–80% of the maximum weight tolerated by the patient in a single contraction during preliminary testing by the physiotherapist.[17 20] A set of 10 repetitions of each exercise is performed three times with a rest period between sets. Two circuit sessions per week are required and provision of small mobile weights allows a third session at home.

All patients complete a circuit of the same exercises (box) with their own individual prescription. The order of exercises is not critical but must be preceded by a five minute conditioning period of stretching exercises designed to prevent muscle, tendon, and ligament injuries.

This type of training does not require heart rate monitoring as the objective is not central cardiovascular conditioning but rather improving strength and endurance of individual muscle groups. The key to a successful outcome lies in the suitability of initial prescription and then physiotherapist guidance, particularly regarding the speed of repetitions and the length of rest periods between the stations. The individual's response in terms of breathlessness is of paramount importance to the physiotherapist. Each patient is taught to use the Borg score for breathlessness (Table 10.1) to guide the intensity and number of repetitions plus rest times. Before commencing each new exercise the Borg score should have returned to less than 3—that is, adequate recovery time is necessary to allow tolerance of the whole range of circuit exercises.

Mobility (conditioning) programme for patients with severe disease

This group of patients will be unable to participate in whole body endurance training or in multigym weight training. The objective must be to reduce the effects of major skeletal muscle deconditioning and loss of function due to enforced inactivity and poor nutritional status. These patients often have difficulty with the most basic of daily tasks such as rising from bed, dressing, moving from room to room, and washing themselves.

The programme is designed to gently restore locomotor function of individual joint muscles, ligaments, and tendons by a series of careful stretching exercises plus gentle repetitions of muscle contraction and relaxation. By exercising each muscle group *in*

Table 10.1   Borg score for measurement of breathlessness

0	Nothing at all
0·5	Very, very slight (just noticeable)
1	Very slight
2	Slight
3	Moderate
4	Somewhat severe
5	Severe
6	
7	Very severe
8	
9	Very, very severe (almost maximal)
10	Maximal

From Burdon *et al.*[21]

isolation and unloaded, breathlessness is minimised as is the risk of musculoskeletal injury. The programme given in the box on pages 204–5 improves individual muscle strength, endurance, and mobility.[22] This contains a range of upper and lower limb movements including simple modifications such as "wall" press ups and sitting stomach muscle exercises to avoid undue breathlessness due to posture—that is, lying flat. The main attraction of such a programme is that it can be performed at home once learned under careful supervision. One physiotherapy session per week should be allocated to instruction of up to 10 patients and four weekly teaching sessions should suffice for each patient followed by home self management of a *daily* 20 minute session thereafter.

Patient selection for programmes

Referral source

At the outset it is advisable to recruit for pulmonary rehabilitation from the pool of patients attending the routine chest clinic. They will already have been assessed, investigated and, hopefully, be receiving optimal medical treatment. It is therefore easier to concentrate on the remaining issues of mobility and psychosocial function of direct relevance to pulmonary rehabilitation. Although general practitioners may eventually wish to have direct access for referral, the chest clinic is initially an important filter guaranteeing

Circuit of conditioning exercises designed to improve patient's strength and mobility

Shoulder shrugging
Circling shoulder girdle forwards, down, backwards and up. Keep timing constant allowing two full seconds per circle. Relaxation encouraged throughout. Continue for 30 seconds. Repeat the exercise three times with short rest intervals between sets until Borg score is less than 3

Full arm circling
One arm at a time, passing arm as near as possible to side of head, circle arm in as large circles as possible. (Allow 8–10 seconds per complete circle.) Repeat for 40 seconds continuously. Repeat the exercise three times with short rest intervals between. Repeat with other arm

Increasing arm circle
Hold arm away from body at shoulder height. Progressively increase size of circle for a count of six circles in 10 seconds then decrease for a further count of six. Repeat for 40 seconds. Repeat with other arm

Abdominal exercise
Sitting in chair, tighten abdominal muscles, hold for a count of four and then release muscles over four seconds to starting position. Repeat continuously for 30 seconds. Perform the procedure three times with short rest periods in between

Wall press ups
Stand with feet a full arm's length distance from wall, place hands on wall and bend at elbow until nose touches the wall, push arms straight again allowing eight seconds approximately from start to completion. Repeat for 40 seconds continuously to a total of five repetitions. Repeat procedure three times with short rest periods in between

Sitting to standing
Using dining room chair, sit, stand, sit allowing 8–10 seconds from start to completion. Repeat continuously for 40 seconds to a total of five repetitions. Perform exercise three times with short rest intervals in between

Quadriceps exercise
Sitting on chair straighten right knee, tense thigh muscle, hold for count of four, then relax gradually over a further four seconds to a total of five repetitions over 40 seconds. Repeat the exercise three times with short rest periods in between. Repeat procedure with left leg

---

Circuit of conditioning exercises designed to improve patient's strength and mobility—*continued*

Calf exercises
Holding on to back of chair, go up on to toes, return to floor taking 8–10 seconds to complete the procedure. Repeat continuously for 40 seconds

Calf alternates/walking on the spot
Holding on to back of chair, allow one knee to bend, keeping toes on the ground. Bend other knee, while straightening first knee and allow four seconds for complete procedure. Repeat this bending/straightening of knees, that is, walking on the spot, keeping toes on the ground continuously for 40 seconds to a total of 10 repetitions. Repeat the exercise three times with short rest periods in between

Step ups
Step up with right foot onto step then bring up left foot. Step down with right foot then left foot. Allow four seconds for the complete procedure and repeat continuously for 40 seconds. Repeat the exercise three times with short rest periods in between

---

appropriate usage of the new facilities, particularly until general practitioners develop the necessary experience of the programme as applied to their patients.

Referral criteria

All patients with COPD are potential candidates for rehabilitation, either for entry to the complete programme or just to specific aspects. There is recent recognition[23] that severe disease is not the only criterion, provided that a range of programme options is available to suit the spectrum of illness severity. Therefore selection should be very carefully made on the basis of:

1 An identifiable problem for which the programme can be expected to provide quantifiable benefit
2 A realistic attitude and understanding on the patient's part of the requirements for a regular commitment during the training period plus the likely benefits and limitations of the programme
3 Availability of places on the programme—that is, on a "first come first serve" basis.

The types of programmes available allow a preliminary streamlining of the selection process. Using the principles outlined in the American Thoracic Society guidelines for evaluation of impairment secondary to respiratory disease[24] we use the following severity gradings to group patients before exercise assessment. Patients with mild COPD have values for FEV_1, FVC, and FEV_1/FVC ratio of more than 60% the normal predicted values, patients with moderate disease have values between 40% and 60% predicted values, and patients with severe disease have values less than 40% predicted and/or T_{LCO} less than 60% predicted. Although the results of exercise evaluation finally determine the choice of programme, these broad categories are helpful in the initial selection process. Patients with mild disease may be considered for the aerobic programme at the outset. Patients with moderate disease are more likely to complete successfully the multigym programme and may then be considered for aerobic training. Patients with severe disease should be referred to the conditioning programme and may then graduate to the multigym programme.

Programme evaluation (medical audit)

Every patient's progress should be carefully documented and an overall assessment of the success rate for each programme in achieving these objectives for the three categories of illness severity should be determined annually. The psychosocial assessments such as the quality of life questionnaires are useful in practical terms—that is, individual patient management—but one should not rely on a single aggregate score to determine the success or failure of the programme for the patient. Individual problems may respond successfully to the programme while the total score is unchanged, and these problems should have been identified as targets in the pulmonary assessment.

Finally, it is also worth considering rather more ambitious targets at the outset such as a reduction in hospital inpatient requirements (a significant financial incentive to the administration) and demands on general practitioner services. Similar programmes in which a patient's progress in the year before pulmonary rehabilitation has been compared with the year after and also with subsequent years have successfully achieved these aims in the United States of America, suggesting that improvements can be maintained in some patients.[25][26] The programme should be viewed primarily as an aid to patient management of his or her illness within the community rather than in hospital.

Continuing care after programme completion

Patients should be reviewed at the pulmonary rehabilitation medical assessment clinic six monthly for two years after programme completion. The objectives are to review progress in achieving targets decided on completion of pulmonary rehabilitation and to provide encouragement to continue. Participation in pulmonary rehabilitation is usually a very positive experience because of improvements in daily functioning and self confidence, and also because of the companionship offered. The challenge is therefore to find a suitable substitute. Self help groups of programme "graduates" are extremely useful and the programme director should be affiliated to the group to encourage its development. The following are suggestions to help the process forward:

1 The hospital may be able to provide a regular meeting venue.
2 Patients should be encouraged to use local authority leisure and fitness centre facilities to continue the programme and to participate in activities such as swimming or bowling. Liaison of the programme physiotherapist with the centre's staff is helpful (these centres may require confirmation that medicolegal responsibility remains with the patient, not the leisure centre, and also that supervision will not be required).
3 Walking in groups is a simple social way of participating in exercise. Our programme has identified several alternative routes adjacent to the hospital with target distances to walk. Patients can also find convenient areas in town centres to walk and then meet socially.
4 Local authorities or voluntary organisations may have a service which can transport patients to meeting points if adequate notice is given.

Consideration of special patient groups

Patients requiring oxygen therapy

In the United Kingdom long term oxygen therapy prescription is covered by existing routine clinical services. The important issue is to determine the patients' requirements for oxygen supplementation during pulmonary rehabilitation exercise programmes. The following steps are necessary:

1 Initial documentation of desaturation during exercise (this should be determined at the initial evaluation in the laboratory or field tests)
2 Oxygen supplementation for these patients during the exercise programmes on the rationale that the potential for cardiac arrhythmias may be reduced and that exercise may be better tolerated.[27]

The conditioning programme for severely disabled patients is the most appropriate choice for these patients at the outset. Although desaturation may not be provoked by this programme on a single occasion, oxygen should be routinely administered as a precaution. A major component, however, is conditioning at home. In the United Kingdom patients do not have access to portable oxygen by NHS prescription and it will be necessary to provide a renewable oxygen cylinder purely for use during the home unsupervised daily sessions where portable oxygen is not feasible on cost grounds. Prescription of oxygen for exercise *outwith* the rehabilitation programme—for example, to allow greater mobility during activities *outside* the home—remains an unresolved problem while there is a lack of guidelines within the United Kingdom.

Patients with illnesses other than COPD

Asthma (see also chapter 11)

Pulmonary rehabilitation has largely been confined to patients with COPD, but there is now a recognition that other patient groups may benefit. The principle of asthma rehabilitation has been discussed in an editorial in *Thorax*,[15] and programmes for exercise rehabilitation in asthma have recently been extensively reviewed.[28] The issues of drug therapy, education, and compliance are covered by the recent international consensus guidelines as fundamental requirements of routine clinical provision, and the application of pulmonary rehabilitation to asthma largely refers to exercise provision. The principles are the same as those described in this chapter with some additional considerations. The nature of the illness is different from COPD, usually affecting younger patients with different expectations. Separation of training sessions is therefore advisable to allow clear and separate goals to be pursued by each group. Patients with mild asthma provide the largest number of subjects and can greatly benefit both by improving cardiorespiratory fitness[27] and by overcoming the fear and inhibition of exercise which is very common.[28-30]

The conditioning programme is a suitable introduction to exercise for steroid dependent asthmatic patients who may then graduate to the other programmes after further assessment. Steroid induced osteoporosis is not a contraindication to exercise which has been shown to be beneficial in slowing progression of the disease.[31]

Interstitial lung disease, cystic fibrosis, and lung transplant recipients

Some experience of pulmonary rehabilitation of these patient groups has been published.[32-34] Aspects such as education, psychosocial counselling, nutritional assessment, and drug and oxygen requirements are inherent parts of optimal management in these conditions. The objective of exercise programmes is to improve mobility. The principles outlined in this chapter apply to lung disease in general and are useful guidelines for specialist units considering commencing exercise programmes for these groups of patients.

Finally, it should be evident that enthusiasm, clear objectives at the outset, and communication particularly with primary care (general practice) are fundamental prerequisites for the successful introduction of a pulmonary rehabilitation programme.

Acknowledgments

I am greatly indebted to my colleagues in the Department of Respiratory Medicine and, in particular, to Mrs Elaine Mackay who is currently implementing the pulmonary rehabilitation programmes discussed in this chapter.

1 Make BJ. Pulmonary rehabilitation: myths or reality. *Clin Chest Med* 1986;7: 519–40.
2 American College of Sports Medicine. *Guidelines for graded exercise testing and exercise prescription,* 3rd edn. Philadelphia: Lea & Febiger, 1990.
3 Gilmartin M. Patient and family education. *Clin Chest Med* 1986;7:619–27.
4 Wasserman K, Hansen JE, Sue DY, Whipp BJ. *Principles of exercise testing and interpretation.* Philadelphia: Lea & Febiger, 1987.

5 Jones NL, Campbell EJM. *Clinical exercise testing*, 2nd edn. Philadelphia: WB Saunders, 1981.

6 Zigmond AS, Snaith RP. The Hospital Anxiety and Depression Scale. *Acta Psychiatr Scand* 1983;**67**:361–70.

7 Eakin P. Assessment of activities of daily living: a critical review. *Br J Occup Ther* 1989;**52**:11–5.

8 Schwarzer R (ed). *Self-efficacy: thought control of action.* Washington DC: Hemisphere, 1992.

9 Donahoe M, Rogers RM. Nutritional assessment and support in chronic obstructive pulmonary disease. *Clin Chest Med* 1990;**11**:499–512.

10 Mancino JM, Donohue M, Rogers RM. Nutritional assessment and therapy. In: Casaburi R, Petty TL (eds), *The principles and practice of pulmonary rehabilitation.* Philadelphia: WB Saunders, 1993.

11 Hughes RL, Davidson R. Limitations of exercise reconditioning in COLD. *Chest* 1983;**83**:241–9.

12 Butland RJA, Gross ER, Pang J, Woodcock AA, Geddes DM. Two-, six-, and 12-minute walking tests in respiratory diseases. *BMJ* 1982;**284**:1607–8.

13 Singh SJ, Morgan MDL, Scott S, Walters D, Hardman E. Development of a shuttle walking test of disability in patients with chronic airways obstruction. *Thorax* 1992;**47**:1019–24.

14 Bruce RA. Exercise testing of patients with coronary artery disease. *Ann Clin Res* 1971;**3**:323–32.

15 Clark CJ. Asthma and exercise: a suitable case for rehabilitation. *Thorax* 1992; **47**:765–7.

16 Simpson K, Killian K, McCartney N, Stubbing DG, Jones NL. Randomised controlled trial of weight lifting exercise in patients with chronic airflow limitation. *Thorax* 1992;**47**:70–5.

17 Astrand PO, Rhodahl K. *Textbook of work physiology*, 2nd edn. New York: McGraw-Hill, 1992.

18 Belman MJ. Exercise in patients with chronic obstructive pulmonary disease. *Thorax* 1993;**48**:936–46.

19 Casaburi R. Exercise training in chronic obstructive lung disease. In: Casaburi R, Petty TL (eds), *The principles and practice of pulmonary rehabilitation.* Philadelphia: WB Saunders, 1993.

20 Brown AB, McCartney N, Sale DG. Positive adaptation to weightlifting training in the elderly. *J Appl Physiol* 1990;**69**:1725–33.

21 Burdon JC, Juniper EF, Killian KJ, Hargreaves FE, Campbell EJM. The perception of breathlessness in asthma. *Am Rev Respir Dis* 1982;**128**:825–8.

22 Mackay E, Cochrane LM, Clark CJ. The effects of sequential isolated muscle training on peripheral muscle conditioning and exercise tolerance in patients with COPD. *Eur Respir J* 1992;**5**(suppl 15):30S.

23 European Respiratory Society Rehabilitation and Chronic Care Scientific Group. Pulmonary rehabilitation in chronic obstructive pulmonary disease (COPD) with recommendations for its use. *Eur Respir Rev* 1991;**6**:1–568.

24 American Thoracic Society. Evaluation of impairment/disability secondary to respiratory disease. *Am Rev Respir Dis* 1982;**1**:945–51.

25 Mall RW, Medeiros M. Objective evaluation of results of a pulmonary rehabilitation programme in a community hospital. *Chest* 1989;**94**:1156–60.

26 Bebout DE, Hodgkin JE, Zorn EG, Yee AR, Sammer EA. Clinical and physiological outcomes of a university-hospital pulmonary rehabilitation programme. *Respir Care* 1983;**28**:1468–73.

27 Patessio A, Iolo F, Donner CF. Exercise prescription. In: Casaburi R, Petty TL (eds), *The principles and practice of pulmonary rehabilitation.* Philadelphia: WB Saunders, 1993.

28 Clark CJ. The role of physical training in asthma. In: Casaburi R, Petty TL (eds), *The principles and practice of pulmonary rehabilitation.* Philadelphia: WB Saunders, 1993.

29 Cochrane LM, Clark CJ. Benefits and problems of a physical training programme for asthmatic patients. *Thorax* 1990;**5**:345–51.

30 Strunk RC, Mrazek DA, Fukuhara JT, Masterton J, Ludwick SK, LaBrecque JF. Cardiovascular fitness in children with asthma correlates with psychological functioning of the child. *Pediatrics* 1989;**26**:2798–86.

31 Weston AR, Macfarlane DJ, Hopkins WG. Physical activity of asthmatic and non-asthmatic children. *J Asthma* 1989;**26**:279–86.

32 Meyer R, Kroner-Herwig B, Sporkel H. The effect of exercise and induced expectations on visceral perception in asthmatic patients. *J Psychosom Res* 1990; **34**:455–60.

33 McLatchie GR. Sport and exercise in the prevention and treatment of disease. In: McLatchie GR, ed. *Essentials of sports medicine,* 2nd edn. London: Churchill Livingstone, 1993.

34 Foster S, Thomas M III. Pulmonary rehabilitation in lung disease other than chronic obstructive pulmonary disease. *Am Rev Respir Dis* 1990;**141**:601–4.

35 Orenstein DM, Noyes BF. Cystic fibrosis. In: Casaburi R, Petty TL (eds), *The principles and practice of pulmonary rehabilitation.* Philadelphia: WB Saunders, 1993.

36 Biggar DG, Malen JF, Trulock EP, Cooper JD. Pulmonary rehabilitation before and after lung transplantation. In: Casaburi R, Petty TL (eds), *The principles and practice of pulmonary rehabilitation.* Philadelphia: WB Saunders, 1993.

11 Pulmonary rehabilitation in non-COPD disorders

AK SIMONDS

The concept of rehabilitation for pulmonary conditions other than chronic obstructive pulmonary disease (COPD) is not new. Exercise regimens to improve health in individuals with chronic tuberculous lung disease have been advocated since Ancient Grecian times and were taken up by the Sanatorium movement in the second half of the nineteenth century. These programmes included graduated walking, hill climbing, and, sometimes, active labour.[1] Although many pulmonary TB patients reported benefit, hazards were also evident—part of the half mile walk at Frimley Sanatorium, England became known as haemorrhage hill. Selection of appropriate patients for rehabilitation remains to this day a key issue, although perhaps for less dramatic reasons.

Many current pulmonary rehabilitation programmes include a training/exercise component, but also incorporate coverage of educational aspects, behavioural techniques, and psychosocial issues. Individuals with chronic pulmonary conditions other than COPD (for example, chest wall disorders, pulmonary fibrosis, bronchiectasis, and asthma) are now routinely admitted to rehabilitation programmes. Information on the outcome of pulmonary rehabilitation in these patients is limited because of the heterogeneous nature of the underlying disorders and small numbers in some subgroups. Widespread rehabilitation programmes for patients with asthma, cystic fibrosis, and those who have received heart/lung transplantation have, however, recently been developed. In addition, new views on the value of exercise versus rest have lead to training programmes for patients with primary neuromuscular disease. In this chapter emphasis will be placed on

212

the training component of pulmonary rehabilitation schemes as this is the area that has received most investigative attention.

Cardiorespiratory responses to exercise

Asthma

Airway narrowing in asthma, as in COPD, has a significant effect on dynamic lung function and the work of breathing. In contrast to COPD patients, individuals with asthma usually show a greater variability in airflow obstruction, and are more susceptible to exercise induced exacerbations. These potential problems necessitate specific rehabilitation strategies.

Pulmonary resistance in asthma is the result of a combination of reduction in airway calibre, an increase in tissue viscosity, and rise in upper airway resistance.[2] Hyperinflation occurs when prolonged emptying of the lungs causes end expiratory volume to excede relaxed volume. Breathlessness in acute asthma is largely attributable to breathing at increased lung volumes rather than resulting from an increase in airway resistance.[3]

If airflow obstruction is mild, impairment in exercise tolerance is unlikely. Usually ventilatory capacity has to be reduced to less than 70% predicted before there is a progressive deleterious effect on exercise performance. In this event, results commonly seen are a low maximum power output and reduced maximum oxygen consumption ($\dot{V}o_2$max), coupled with ventilation at peak exercise which is close to maximal voluntary ventilation (MVV). In severe airflow obstruction, expiratory airflow is limited by maximum flow–volume characteristics and a situation is reached where an increase in respiratory frequency is accompanied by a fall in tidal volume (V_T). Hypercapnia on exercise occurs if there is a high dead space (V_D) to tidal volume ratio ($V_T:V_D$), or more rarely in situations where there is coexistent respiratory muscle weakness/fatigue, or an abnormality of central ventilatory drive.

Pulmonary fibrosis

Diffuse alveolitis results in a greater reduction in maximum power output and $\dot{V}o_2$max than airflow obstruction when associated with a similar level of impairment in ventilatory capacity.[4] In moderate to severe interstitial lung disease, ventilation is excessive at all levels of exercise and reaches ventilatory capacity earlier via

213

a low V_T, high frequency pattern accompanied by ventilation–perfusion mismatch. Lactic acid production may occur at relatively low levels of exercise as a result of hypoxaemia, although circulatory factors may contribute as a result of additional pulmonary vascular disease. The degree of hypoxaemia on exercise cannot be predicted easily by resting arterial oxygen tensions or saturation. It is therefore important to monitor arterial oxygen saturation during exercise.

Chest wall disorders

Several studies have examined the factors leading to respiratory impairment in scoliotic individuals. Multivariate analysis[5] in young adults with adolescent onset scoliosis has shown that the severity of the scoliosis (as measured by the angle of curvature and number of vertebrae involved), a high dorsal location of the curve, and loss of thoracic kyphosis all contribute significantly to a reduction in vital capacity. The duration of the curvature, degree of spinal rotation, and respiratory muscle strength were not found to be correlated with pulmonary function. It should, however, be noted that respiratory muscle strength in these adolescents was not significantly reduced (maximum expiratory pressure, MEP, 81% predicted; maximum inspiratory pressure, MIP, 78% predicted). By contrast, respiratory muscle function is likely to be a major determinant of pulmonary function in adults with primary neuromuscular disease affecting the respiratory muscles. In addition, although the specific age of onset does not appear to influence lung volumes in those who develop a curvature in adolescence, a longitudinal study[6] has shown that patients who acquire a scoliosis before the age of five years are at high risk of cardiorespiratory decompensation later in life. Those with adolescent onset curves appear to be at low risk, unless there is additional pulmonary pathology (for example, smoking induced chronic airflow obstruction), or vital capacity is less than 50% predicted at presentation.

Kearon et al[7] have investigated the clinical features that determine exercise tolerance in adolescent idiopathic scoliosis. Work capacity in 79 subjects (age 21 ± 10 years, mean vital capacity 78% predicted) was measured using an incremental cycle test. Compared with normals, the work capacity of the scoliotic subjects was 86% (81·9–89·7%) predicted, with $\dot{V}O_2max$ 76% predicted. Both ventilatory impairment and peripheral muscle function influenced work capacity. A high heart rate response at submaximal work rates was also predictive of reduced work capacity. The authors concluded that the reduced work capacity and resulting disability in these mildly affected individuals (mean angle of curvature 45°) results from a combination of decreased ventilatory capacity, reduced muscularity, and cardiorespiratory deconditioning.

Fitness in non-COPD respiratory disorders

A sedentary lifestyle with limited exposure to exercise are well established features of COPD. Lack of fitness is also an important factor in non-COPD patients. In children and young adults with asthma, cystic fibrosis, chest wall disorders, and neuromuscular disease, exercise is often discouraged in infancy, leading to a lifelong fear of exertion which may be misguidedly reinforced by parents, teachers, and medical advisers. Individuals with chest wall deformity may also avoid swimming and sporting activities because of self consciousness about their body shape.

Asthma

Despite educational initiatives, teachers of sports and physical education feel inadequately prepared to supervise asthmatic children.[8] There is room for improvement in encouraging staff to recommend the use of β_2 agonists before exercise and to select sporting activities that are less likely to provoke exercise induced asthma. On a psychosomatic level it has been pointed out that the anticipation of "harmful" breathlessness can enhance the subject's perception of the "cost" of exercise which may, in turn, affect airway resistance.[9] Similar influences may operate in chest wall disease and patients with cystic fibrosis.

Considering the reduced level of participation in sporting activities, it is not surprising that most studies that have assessed fitness levels in asthmatic subjects have demonstrated suboptimal exercise capability. The interpretation of the results of these studies of fitness is limited by the fact that many do not include controls or indicate whether pre-treatment with bronchodilators was given.[10] Reasonably representative results, however, show that in 65 children with moderate to severe asthma, 50% were severely deconditioned.[11] There was no correlation between the severity of airflow obstruction and level of fitness. In another study[12] three quarters of asthmatic children scored below the 25th percentile of

215

a normal range established by a nine minute run in a field study of age matched controls.

In a comparison of 44 young asthmatic adults with 64 controls who did not exercise regularly, Cochrane and Clark[13] showed that the asthmatic group had a lower mean oxygen consumption and reduced anaerobic threshold, but there was no difference in maximum heart rate between the groups, indicating that the main limitation to exercise for both groups was cardiovascular rather than ventilatory. A measure of dyspnoea, maximum minute ventilation as a percentage of maximum voluntary ventilation ($\dot{V}$Emax/MVV), was higher in asthmatic subjects at maximum exercise rate, and at the submaximal workload level which produced 75% of the maximum heart rate. No relationship was, however, found between FEV_1 (pre- or postbronchodilator) and $\dot{V}O_2$max, anaerobic threshold or O_2 pulse (defined as $\dot{V}O_2$max per heart beat). This study convincingly demonstrates that asthma did not limit the performance of high intensity exercise and that factors other than airflow obstruction are the main determinants of exercise limitation.

Cystic fibrosis

Freeman et al[14] have compared maximum exercise and endurance exercise capacity in patients with cystic fibrosis and matched control subjects. The cystic fibrosis group had a wide range of lung function with FEV_1 between 24% and 117% predicted. Maximum workload and $\dot{V}O_2$max were reduced in patients with cystic fibrosis, with a correlation between disease severity and $\dot{V}O_2$max. Maximum exercise capacity was correlated with percentage body fat (as an indicator of nutritional status), although the addition of this factor in multiple regression analysis did not further explain the reduction in $\dot{V}O_2$max.

The endurance capacity of the patients with cystic fibrosis at the same percentage of $\dot{V}O_2$max did not differ from the control group and this value was not correlated with maximal exercise capacity, lung function, or nutritional status.

Additional work has confirmed that patients with cystic fibrosis with near normal lung function have normal exercise abilities, whereas those with severe impairment of pulmonary function, as expected, do less well. Women with cystic fibrosis have a lower exercise capability than men.[15] Despite the broad correlation between disease severity and exercise ability, pulmonary function is a poor predictor of exercise tolerance on an individual basis, because there is wide intersubject variability. Within individuals, however, improvement in lung function following an acute infective exacerbation is associated with an increase in $\dot{V}O_2$max and a lower perception of exertion at higher work rates.[16]

Maximum heart rate is rarely achieved in moderate to severe cystic fibrosis, because ventilatory factors limit exercise before this peak is reached. In severely affected individuals cardiac stroke volume as a percentage of the predicted value is correlated with resting PO_2, FEV_1, and respiratory duty cycle, indicating a mechanical level of cardiopulmonary interdependence. Stroke volume has been shown to be reduced in 13 poorly nourished patients with cystic fibrosis compared with nine who had a good nutritional status.[17]

It is important to note that exercise tolerance in cystic fibrosis has been shown to be correlated with quality of life indices and survival.[18]

Pulmonary transplant candidates

Assessment and rehabilitation programmes for candidates for single lung, double lung, and heart/lung transplantation have developed rapidly over the past five years as transplant activity has increased. Lung transplant recipients usually have COPD or interstitial lung disease. Preoperative exercise testing in these patients shows very limited exercise performance, and nearly all desaturate on exertion. Patients awaiting transplantation cite leg discomfort, fatigue, and dyspnoea as the main limiting factors.[19] Here too, muscle deconditioning is inevitably present. In patients with severe end stage lung disease, weight loss is common and associated with high respiratory muscle demands. Nutritional supplementation in these circumstances seems sensible. In individuals with interstitial lung disease, dyspnoea is the main cause of exercise limitation.

Following single lung transplantation, FEV_1 and FVC usually increase to 50% predicted, with a PO_2 in excess of 10 kPa (75 mm Hg) and oxygen diffusing capacity (DLCO) of more than 70% predicted. No difference in outcome is seen following right or left single lung transplantation. After double lung or heart/lung transplantation, lung volumes increase to 80–100% predicted, although interestingly there may be no difference between single lung and double lung transplant recipients for 3–24 weeks.[20] It has been postulated[19] that circulatory factors limiting $\dot{V}O_2$max, heart

217

rate, and pulse oximetry may continue to operate post-transplantation. Exercise tends to be terminated by the patient because of fatigue or leg tiredness, indicating continued deconditioning in the face of normalising spirometry. This is unsurprising as most transplant recipients have suffered several years of progressive decline and immobility and are recovering from a major surgical insult.

By way of confirmation, Lonsdorfer and colleagues[21] found that peripheral muscle limitation is the dominant factor in heart transplant recipients. Peripheral muscle ultrasonographic studies before and after a six week training programme in recipients showed an increase in mitochondrial volume density and a preferential expansion in subsarcolemmal mitochondria and intracellular lipid, consistent with increased aerobic capacity of the muscle. Muscle capillary density did not alter, suggesting that changes in perfusion are a more delayed response. In these studies lactate was the main determinant of ventilatory drive resulting from increased reliance on anaerobic mechanisms. A similar effect occurs in unfit sedentary normals.[22]

Interstitial lung disease

Burdon *et al*[23] studied the response to exercise using cycle ergonometry in 41 patients with pulmonary fibrosis in whom vital capacity was reduced on average to 62% predicted. Compared with matched controls, the pulmonary fibrosis patients achieved 53% maximum power output. Both maximum ventilation and maximum power output were linearly related to vital capacity. Arterial oxygen saturation fell by more than 5% in around a third of patients, but there was no correlation between the degree of desaturation and total lung capacity (TLC) or vital capacity (VC). In addition to a reduction in power output, those with a greater impairment in lung volume showed a higher ventilatory response to exercise as a consequence of desaturation and high V_D/V_T ratio. An analysis of the pattern and timing of breathing demonstrated that V_T was reduced in proportion to VC ($r = 0.76$), but that, at low VC levels, V_T was higher in pulmonary fibrosis patients than control subjects with a similar VC. T_{TOT} (total respiratory cycle time) fell during exercise in patients and controls, but T_{TOT} for specific levels of ventilation was shorter in patients, as was inspiratory duration (T_I) and T_I/T_{TOT}. It is clear that pulmonary

218

fibrosis adds to the elastic load on the inspiratory muscles. To cope with the increase in demands incurred by exercise, peak inspiratory force and duration of force development are reduced which may delay the onset of fatigue.

A few individuals with marked desaturation (Sao_2 fall of >20%) were able to achieve high power outputs. In this situation increased cardiac output may be sufficient to maintain peripheral oxygen delivery. The presence of pulmonary hypertension will, however, reduce the cardiac response to exercise. A low stroke volume, high heart rate response was shown in a small number of patients with severe pulmonary impairment, producing a marked reduction in power output. Falls in Sao_2 occurred in this subgroup, but were insufficient to explain the heart rate increase, suggesting that an impaired stroke volume response to exercise was responsible.

The effects of exercise in individuals with milder forms of interstitial lung disease have been examined in sarcoidosis patients with normal spirometry.[24] Patients were divided into those with normal diffusing capacity for carbon monoxide ($Tlco$) (group A) and those with reduced $Tlco$ (group B). A peak $\dot{V}o_2$ of more than 75% predicted was achieved in 86% of group A and 56% of group B. Increased dead space (Vd/Vt) and widening of alveolar–arterial gradient on exercise was seen in a third of group A and most of group B. Half of group A demonstrated excessive ventilation on exercise, and this was a universal finding in group B. These results confirm that, in patients with pulmonary sarcoidosis who have normal spirometry and normal $Tlco$, abnormalities of ventilation occur on exercise in around half, usually associated with a high Vd/Vt ratio. A reduction in $Tlco$ is predictive of an increased frequency of abnormal exercise response, including desaturation.

Chest wall disorders

$\dot{V}o_2$max is lower in scoliotic patients than in controls, with the exception of young patients with a mild deformity (for example, Cobb angle 12–40°) in whom $\dot{V}o_2$max and ventilation have been shown to be normal.[25] In a study of adults with mild to moderate idiopathic thoracic curves (Cobb angle 25–70°, mean vital capacity 81% predicted), Kesten et al[26] demonstrated a significant decrease in $\dot{V}o_2$max compared with age and sex matched controls. Indices of ventilation such as the Vtmax/VC ratio and the dyspnoea index were similar to corresponding values in normals. Hypercapnic and hypoxic ventilatory responses were also within the normal range, indicating that impairment in exercise performance in mild to moderate scoliosis cannot be attributed to ventilatory limitation, but is the result of a reduction in cardiorespiratory fitness.

An analysis of individuals with scoliosis of varying aetiology and variable but mainly severe scoliosis (vital capacity of $0 \cdot 5$–$2 \cdot 95$ litres, Cobb angle of 20–130°), also showed that $\dot{V}o_2$ was reduced compared with age matched controls. Here $\dot{V}o_2$ was proportional to FEV_1 and maximum exercise ventilation.[27] Minute ventilation was increased by around 20%. Heart rate increases were greater than predicted, but this result and the reduction in $\dot{V}o_2$ may be partly related to the fact that a number of subjects had poliomyelitis resulting in a low functional muscle bulk.

Shneerson[28] measured the effects of exercise while breathing air or oxygen in 25 adults with scoliosis. Pulmonary artery mean pressure at rest was $19 \cdot 8$ mm Hg and rose to $35 \cdot 8$ mm Hg on exercise. In 17 subjects pulmonary artery pressure during exertion exceeded 40 mm Hg. Mean pulmonary artery pressure (PAP) increased linearly with $\dot{V}o_2max$ and work rate. Importantly, the rate of rise of PAP as a function of $\dot{V}o_2max$ was inversely related to lung volumes (vital capacity, total lung capacity, and functional residual capacity), and *not* related to Pao_2, or the level and extent of the scoliosis. This effect—of a restricted pulmonary vascular bed causing pulmonary hypertension on exercise in the absence of hypoxaemia—was seen exclusively in individuals with a vital capacity of less than one litre. Breathing 100% oxygen lowered resting PAP and PAP after exercise by a trivial amount, but had little effect on the significant rise in PAP *during* exercise.

Neuromuscular disease

The effects of exercise and muscle training in patients with neuromuscular disease have not been widely studied. There are interesting data on paraplegic and quadriplegic wheelchair athletes, but concerns about the deleterious consequences of exercise on dystrophic muscle, plus the possible overuse of compensatory muscle groups and the risks of associated coexistent cardiomyopathy, have tended to restrict investigation.

Lyager *et al*[29] looked at the cardiorespiratory response to exercise in adults with muscular dystrophy and spinal muscular atrophy. There was no difference between patients and normals in O_2

uptake/pulse per kg body weight. Patients, however, had a higher heart rate response.

Cardiovascular fitness is an important quality of life issue in those with stable non-progressive neuromuscular disease, for example, caused by established spinal injury. Evidence from multiple regression studies suggests that variables such as aerobic power, body mass index, and lung function are major influences on increased productivity across a range of work, educational, and leisure activities. For optimal mobility, individuals need to meet the energy demands of propelling a wheelchair and, if ambulation is possible, this may require a greater energy expenditure than needed for a normal gait.

There are specific concerns regarding the physiological response to exercise in those with spinal injuries, such as a reduction in venous preloading caused by venous pooling. Lesions at T5 produce loss of venous tone in the upper and lower limbs; sympathetic innervation to the legs is lost in lesions below T10. Above T4 cardiac sympathetic tone is absent, resulting in an absence of chronotropic and inotropic responses. Diaphragm function is compromised in lesions proximal to C5.

Assessing cardiorespiratory function in those who cannot carry out standard ergonometry creates its own problems. Wheelchair and arm crank ergonometers can, however, be used. Shepard[30] describes a basic assessment of aerobic status by measuring the maximum distance covered during 12 minutes of manual wheelchair ambulation. Clearly this is difficult to standardise due to variation in wheelchairs, and differences in seating and floor material. In addition, not all neuromuscular patients use a wheelchair and in those who do, arm and leg weakness may be asymmetrical, for example, in poliomyelitis.

During wheelchair exercise the heart is subject to a substantial increase in afterload from upper arm activity, together with the possible loss of inotropic and chronotropic cardiac reflexes. For this reason, initial careful monitoring of heart rhythm plus ST changes is mandatory. The sitting position also compromises respiratory muscle function in some subjects and this may be a particular problem in those with a scoliosis. It is worth bearing in mind that smoking is more common in wheelchair dependent individuals than normal people and will increase the degree of cardiorespiratory risk. Advice regarding smoking cessation is clearly as relevant in some non-COPD groups as in standard COPD programmes.

221

Outcome of rehabilitation programmes

General

Around 10% of patients admitted to pulmonary rehabilitation programmes have conditions other than COPD. Foster and Thomas[31] have reported their experience with a group of non-obstructive lung disease patients, and compared the outcome of these subjects with a COPD group who underwent an identical regimen. Out of a total of 32 non-COPD patients recruited over four years, seven had pulmonary fibrosis, seven bronchiectasis, eight chest wall disorders, four neuromuscular disease, and seven miscellaneous (post adult respiratory distress syndrome or lung resection). On entry to the programme, mean (SD) vital capacity was 1·2 (0·45) litres, FEV_1 0·88 (0·3) litre, PImax 39 (22) cm H_2O, PEmax 43 (23) cm H_2O, Pao_2 8·9 (1·6) kPa, $Paco_2$ 5·7 (1·1) kPa. The four week *inpatient* exercise regimen consisted of two 45 minute physical therapy sessions per day, one occupational therapy session with daily education, and relaxation classes. Educational content was tailored to individual requirements. After four weeks significant improvements in six minute walk, PEmax, and Pao_2 were seen. The greatest increment was found in those with fibrothorax, and the least improvement in patients with scoliosis (Figure 11·1), although numbers are too small to draw firm conclusions. The benefits were comparable to those seen in COPD patients.

Asthma

If children and adults with asthma are deconditioned can this process be safely reversed by an exercise programme? In 23 asthmatic children and adolescents enrolled on a four month outpatient exercise programme consisting of walking/jogging, work tolerance and peak Vo_2 improved significantly and heart rate at a given submaximal load (60 watts) decreased compared with a control group who did not exercise regularly.[32] β_2 Agonists were given before all exercise sessions. Five subjects experienced mild wheezing during 5–10 of 48 exercise sessions. All episodes of exercise induced asthma were controlled by slowing running to a walking pace. Six individuals in the exercise group versus four in the control group developed exacerbations of asthma during the

222

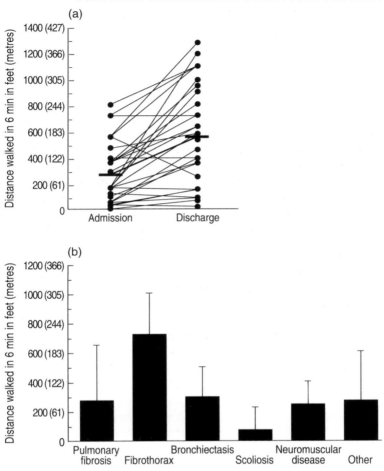

Figure 11.1 (a) Admission and discharge six minute walk distance following pulmonary rehabilitation in 32 non-COPD patients (see text). Improvement in distance walked was significant ($p<0.001$). (b) Increase in six minute walk distance following pulmonary rehabilitation, classified by diagnostic group. Although trends are evident, there was no difference between groups when analysed by ANOVA. (Reproduced with permission from Foster and Thomas.[31])

four month study period; most of these were associated with an upper respiratory tract infection and were not precipitated by an exercise session. Nickerson and colleagues[33] have shown a similar increase in work tolerance, but no improvement in $\dot{V}O_2$max. In

223

this study, no pre-treatment with a β_2 agonist was given and the training period was shorter (six weeks). Orenstein[32] has suggested that the lack of pre-treatment may have limited the attainment of the exercise intensity necessary to increase cardiopulmonary fitness. This impression has been confirmed in children with more severe asthma.[11] Cardiopulmonary fitness was improved in nearly all subjects (38 of 40). Interestingly this gain was achieved over a wide range of baseline performance (Figure 11.2), indicating that the most important factors are the duration and intensity of the training, not the extent of the underlying disease. All children in this study received pre-exercise bronchodilator, and no adverse effects were seen. Not one of these trials, however, includes an assessment of the impact of improved cardiorespiratory fitness on quality of life, school attendance, etc. The authors attributed the substantial improvement in cardiorespiratory fitness to the high intensity inpatient regimen, and the fact that training *and* testing were carried out on a bicycle ergonometer, that is, measurements were exercise specific.

There have been numerous studies of exercise training in adults with asthma; few are controlled, however, and, just as in the case of the paediatric studies, in many bronchodilator pre-treatment is either not given or undocumented. Despite these limitations, there are reassuringly few reports of exercise induced asthma. It should be noted that there is minimal evidence of a change in FEV_1 or peak flow as a result of any pulmonary training regimen.

Cochrane and Clark[13] carried out a controlled three month outpatient programme in adults with moderate asthma (mean FEV_1 2·58 l, 76% predicted). The training schedule consisted of three 30 minute indoor sessions per week. An age matched control group attended the educational sessions, but not the training component of the rehabilitation scheme.

A small improvement in FEV_1 was seen but this did not differ between controls and the training group, and histamine PC_{20} was unaltered. The training group, however, showed significant increases in $\dot{V}o_2$max, maximum O_2 pulse, and anaerobic threshold. $\dot{V}$Emax increased primarily by a rise in $\dot{V}$T, there being little change in respiratory rate or dyspnoea index. At submaximal exercise, lactate level was reduced and $\dot{V}o_2$max increased at most Borg dyspnoea levels. The factors that best predicted the percentage change in $\dot{V}o_2$max were motivation (as judged by attendance record and the assessment of a medical supervisor), initial level of fitness, and symptom score on training days. It was notable that FEV_1

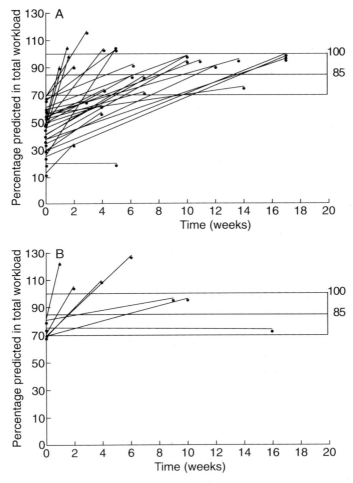

Figure 11.2 Improvement in bicycle ergonometry from admission to post training values in subjects with asthma. Group A had baseline values >2 standard deviations below mean at baseline; group B had values between 1 and 2 standard deviations from mean at baseline. Although rate of improvement varies widely even severely affected children show marked gains. (Reproduced with permission from Ludwick et al.[11])

during the study period, coefficient of variation in peak flow and symptom score, total time spent exercising in hospital, and the number of home sessions all had no independent effect on the change in $\dot{V}o_2$max.

Cystic fibrosis

In an early study Orenstein et al[34] investigated cardiorespiratory fitness, respiratory muscle endurance, and pulmonary function in cystic fibrosis patients with mild pulmonary disease (FEV_1 61% predicted) who underwent a three month running exercise programme. Peak $\dot{V}o_2$, work capacity, and respiratory muscle endurance all improved; pulmonary function was unchanged. No increase in exercise tolerance or cardiorespiratory fitness was seen in the control group. The authors found that it was impossible to predict the extent of improvement from baseline pulmonary function or an initial exercise test, as has been found to be the case in other respiratory disorders.

By contrast, jogging three times a week for 10–30 minutes over eight weeks, in a controlled study carried out by Braggion et al,[35] produced no change in any indices of cardiorespiratory fitness or lung function. Subjects in this study had mild disease and were not markedly deconditioned, indicating that either improvement was not possible, or that the programme was not of sufficient intensity.

Swimming programmes (Casaburi) have produced conflicting results. Zach et al[36] encouraged cystic fibrosis patients to swim for one hour two to three times a week for seven weeks. In another regimen,[37] patients swam three times a week for an initial period of five minutes at 60–75% of maximum heart rate. As an illustration of the variability in results, FEV_1, FVC, peak flow rates, and Schwachmann score (a clinical index of cystic fibrosis health status) were improved in the second study but unchanged in the study of Zach et al.

In a British pulmonary rehabilitation scheme, Webb and colleagues[38] showed that 10 minutes of high intensity work on a cycle ergometer each day over a two week period produced a significant increase in $\dot{V}o_2$max, peak work capacity, and maximum voluntary ventilation. Twelve of 19 patients completed this domiciliary programme. In general, unsupervised home based programmes have lower compliance rates than outpatient schemes—indeed one team has concluded that unsupervised programmes are unlikely to be successful.[39] This impression is, however, contradicted by recent results from a COPD home rehabilitation scheme.[40]

Specific programmes targeted at the respiratory muscles and upper limb muscles have also been assessed in cystic fibrosis. Keens *et al*[41] attempted to train the respiratory muscles using eucapnic hyperpnoeic breathing exercises for 25 minutes a day, five days a week for four weeks. Results showed that the period of sustainable hyperpnoea increased, but it is difficult to know whether this effect translates into a worthwhile gain for the patient, and similar results have been produced by swimming and canoeing. A four week period of inspiratory resistance training[42] resulted in increased inspiratory muscle strength and endurance, but bicycle ergonometry performance did not improve, suggesting that the respiratory muscles are not necessarily the limiting factor in cystic fibrosis. Supportive information comes from an examination of respiratory muscle strength in young adults with moderately severe cystic fibrosis in whom maximum inspiratory and expiratory pressures were shown to be relatively well preserved.[43] A six month weightlifting programme designed to strengthen upper body muscle groups produced an increase in body weight and upper body strength, and reduced hyperinflation, perhaps as a result of increasing chest wall mobility.[44]

Interstitial lung disease

There are few reports of the outcome of exercise programmes in interstitial lung disease. Novitch and Thomas[45] describe experience with two patients with pulmonary fibrosis (one systemic scleroderma, one post acute respiratory distress syndrome) who were able to increase their exercise tolerance markedly after enrolment in an inpatient rehabilitation programme. Both were acutely unwell at the start of the programme, following a period of intensive care, and it is difficult to judge the contribution of exercise training in these non-steady state conditions. However, the same authors have recently reviewed[46] the outcome of pulmonary rehabilitation in 23 patients with pulmonary fibrosis (14 idiopathic pulmonary fibrosis, four sarcoidosis, two interstitial pneumonitis, two scleroderma, and one radiation fibrosis), mean age 65 years. Initial FVC was 1·71 ($50 \pm 21\%$ predicted), DLCO $29 \pm 21\%$ predicted and Pao$_2$ $8·4 \pm 2·5$ kPa (63 ± 19 mm Hg). Six minute walk distance, bicycling time, arm ergonometry, and stair climbing all improved significantly, with mean (SD) six minute walk distance more than doubling from 315 (345) to 719 (537) feet. There was no control group, but the improvement was similar to that achieved by COPD patients taking part in the same programme. Other rehabilitation centres have experienced less encouraging results with interstitial lung disease patients. It is likely that patient selection and the introduction of rehabilitation earlier in the natural history of the condition will be principal determinants of outcome in this group.

Neuromuscular disease

As ventilatory failure resulting from respiratory muscle weakness is an end stage feature of many neuromuscular conditions, much attention has been focused on the benefits and limitations of training the respiratory muscles in this population. Nevertheless, the issue of exercise training is controversial because, although exercise has been shown to be of benefit in some situations, overwork may lead to muscle fatigue and overt tissue damage.[47] Unfortunately many studies have been uncontrolled and/or rely on simple voluntary measurements of global respiratory muscle strength before and after intervention.

Gross et al[48] looked at the effects of resistive breathing in six C3–T1 quadriplegic subjects with vital capacities of between 8% and 48% predicted. An inspiratory resistive load was applied via a Hans–Rudolf valve for 30 minutes a day, six days a week for eight weeks. A progressive increase in both muscle strength and endurance was reported, although the use of the high/low ratio of electromyograph signal to assess fatigue is questionable. To see whether respiratory muscle training would reduce pulmonary complications in young adults with neuromuscular disease, Estrup and colleagues[49] used a four week home programme of maximum inspiratory manoeuvres and resistance breathing in 12 patients with either progressive muscular dystrophy or spinal muscular atrophy types II and III and six normal controls. Mean initial values for the patient group were vital capacity 67% predicted (range 24–108%), MIP 31 cm H_2O, MEP 40 cm H_2O. Five out of nine patients increased their vital capacity on the programme, but there was no change in mouth pressures. Maximum voluntary ventilation (MVV) increased in both patients and controls. Interestingly, a trial of intermittent positive pressure hyperinflation in scoliotic patients, including some with a neuromuscular disease, also produced an increase in vital capacity and MVV,[50] suggesting that passive or active hyperinflation may enhance pulmonary or chest wall compliance.

As training may potentially cause harm in neuromuscular disease, the ability to predict which individuals are likely to benefit would be valuable. This issue has been addressed by a controlled study of inspiratory muscle training in Duchenne muscular dystrophy.[51] Thirty patients took part, with half randomised to training and the other half acting as controls. A specially developed resistive training device was used which provided visual feedback and triggered a videogame on completion of the programme to increase motivation. The training consisted of ten loaded breathing cycles at 70% of maximum transdiaphragmatic pressure carried out twice a day in the home for six months. The level of resistance was increased stepwise during the trial if patients became able to sustain higher pressures. Inspiratory muscle strength was assessed serially using maximal sniff oesophageal and transdiaphragmatic pressures. In 10 of 15 subjects inspiratory muscle strength and endurance were increased significantly after one month, and improved further at three and six months (Figure 11.3). After discontinuation of the programme, improvement was maintained for at least six months, whereas there was no difference in inspiratory muscle parameters in the control group. Lung volumes, 12 second MVV, and Pao_2 were, however, unaltered in both patients and controls. Five of the

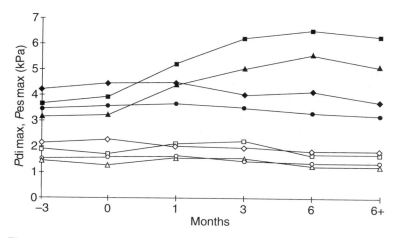

Figure 11.3 Maximal sniff oesophageal (Poesmax) and transdiaphragmatic (Pdimax) values before, during and after respiratory muscle training in 10 subjects who completed training (T), in five subjects with severe pulmonary impairment who discontinued training after one month (T'), in 12 controls without training (C), and three controls with severe pulmonary impairment (C'). ■, Pdimax, T; □, Pdimax, T'; ◆, Pdimax, C; ◇, Pdimax, C'; ▲, Pesmax, T; △, Pesmax, T'; ●, Pesmax, C; ○, Pesmax, C'. (Reproduced with permission from Wanke et al.[50])

training patients withdrew after one month when no increase in muscle function was seen. These five individuals all had a vital capacity of less than 25% predicted and were hypercapnic at the start of the trial. The lack of improvement in the most severely compromised subgroup may indicate that the training intensity was too great. There was, however, no change in creatinine phosphokinase (CPK) levels during the study, suggesting that muscle damage did not occur.

An alternative explanation, as pointed out by the authors, is that end stage Duchenne dystrophy patients may not have sufficient functional muscle to take advantage of a training effect. Overall, several conclusions can be drawn from this study. First, specific inspiratory muscle training may be beneficial in Duchenne muscular dystrophy providing it is introduced early in the natural history of the disease before the onset of ventilatory failure, and second the use of reward devices such as a videogame may improve compliance. These results justify further careful evaluation of training programmes in primary neuromuscular disease.

Practical issues in planning an exercise programme

Possible problems associated with exercise need to be considered before mounting a programme. This means that in many situations the exercise regimen should be tailored to the individual, having carried out a full initial assessment of the severity of the underlying disorder, current therapy, and baseline exercise capability.

There are several practical points that are worth attention (box).

Components of a pulmonary rehabilitation programme in non-COPD patients

The assessment of the outcome of pulmonary rehabilitation in COPD is still in its infancy, although much work is currently being carried out. There are even greater gaps in our knowledge of the outcome and ideal composition of pulmonary rehabilitation programmes for non-COPD patients. For example, there have been no randomised controlled studies of pulmonary rehabilitation in chest wall disorders, interstitial lung disease, and many neuromuscular conditions. Information is accumulating on patients with asthma, cystic fibrosis, and following lung transplantation.

Practical aspects of pulmonary rehabilitation in non-COPD patients

- Self management is an essential component of any rehabilitation programme, but has particular relevance to asthma and cystic fibrosis patients. Advice regarding pre-treatment with bronchodilator to reduce exercise induced asthma and about selection of indoor activities in cold weather is clearly important

- Thermoregulation may be a problem in individuals with cystic fibrosis and quadriplegics with impaired sympathetic innervation. Care should be taken to maintain hydration and avoid overheating. Patients tend to underestimate their fluid needs[51]

- Supplemental oxygen should be used to maintain Sao_2 during exercise. It is helpful to monitor saturation during the initial exercise assessment. Although hypercapnia has not been shown to be a bar to obtaining benefit through rehabilitation in COPD patients,[5] significant hypercapnia in patients with neuromuscular and chest wall disease indicates the need for careful assessment and the consideration of additional management strategies such as non-invasive respiratory support. Hypercapnia in interstitial lung disease is usually an end stage feature, and exercise in this situation may be inadvisable

This chapter has focused on the exercise component of rehabilitation schemes. As with COPD patients, deconditioning is a feature that is likely to exacerbate disability, handicap, and social limitation in non-COPD groups with chronic respiratory disease. Exercise programmes have been shown to be beneficial in some situations (asthma, cystic fibrosis), but large controlled studies are limited. Patients with a wide range of pulmonary function are often included in studies, making it difficult to assess the impact of exercise at different stages of the natural history of a condition. In addition, the intensity of the exercise employed often varies considerably, and details on compliance are commonly omitted. Importantly, even though $\dot{V}o_2$max may improve, the translation of this effect into everyday performance is unknown.

The role of respiratory muscle training is unclear. In COPD the addition of respiratory muscle training to general exercise conditioning produced a 24% increase in maximal workload on a bicycle ergometer, compared with a 12% increase using an exercise conditioning programme alone. It is not known whether this finding is relevant to non-COPD patients in whom respiratory muscles may be significantly weaker. The type of respiratory muscle training used (for example, inspiratory resistance versus normocapnic hyperpnoea) is likely to be crucial. A meta-analysis of respiratory muscle training in COPD found little overall benefit, but did suggest that resistance training during which the breathing pattern is controlled to generate a rise in inspiratory pressure warrants further investigation.[53]

Behavioural aspects have not been assessed in detail. A controlled trial[54] of dyspnoea management in COPD (including teaching of relaxation techniques, breathing retraining, pacing, and panic control) showed, however, that this approach was not helpful as stand alone therapy, but it is possible that dyspnoea management strategies may be of value as adjuncts in other conditions such as interstitial lung disease.

Future research

Pulmonary rehabilitation has recently been the subject of a National Institutes of Health (NIH) workshop.[55] The resulting recommendations include the need for large controlled studies to look at the outcome of pulmonary rehabilitation in terms of mortality, morbidity, physiological indices, hospital admissions, quality of life, and cost effectiveness. In addition, it is clearly important to investigate the transfer of effects of such a programme to the patient's experience of dyspnoea, his or her ability to complete activities of daily living, and the incidence of pulmonary complications. As an interesting angle on exercise relevant to daily life, Ambrosino et al[56] have used simulated daily activities (for example, ironing, sweeping) as a part of a rehabilitation programme and shown that task specific exercise is well tolerated and may improve work capacity without an increase in cardiovascular stress or breathlessness.

Pulmonary rehabilitation in non-COPD is largely uncharted territory and is ripe for investigation. In view of the small numbers of patients with some chronic respiratory disorders, multicentre studies will be required. Children with asthma and cystic fibrosis have been included in pulmonary rehabilitation outcome studies, but improved methods to assess the quality of life in these younger age groups are needed. In particular, the cost effectiveness of inpatient versus outpatient rehabilitation schemes demands close examination.

1 Bignall JR (ed). Graduated labour. In: *Frimley: the biography of a sanatorium.* London: Board of Governors National Heart & Chest Hospital, 1979:30–44.
2 Martin JG. Respiratory mechanics in asthma. *Eur Respir Rev* 1993;3:444–7.
3 Permutt S. Breathlessness in acute asthma. In: Jones NL, Killian KJ (eds), *Breathlessness. The Campbell Symposium.* Canada: Boehringer-Ingelheim Inc, 1992:60–5.
4 Jones NL. Exercise tests. In: Clark TJH (ed), *Clinical investigation of respiratory disease.* London: Chapman & Hall, 1981:95–115.
5 Kearon C, Guillermo RV, Kirkly A, Killian KJ. Factors determining pulmonary function in adolescent idiopathic thoracic scoliosis. *Am Rev Respir Dis* 1993; 148:288–94.
6 Branthwaite MA. Cardiorespiratory consequences of unfused idiopathic scoliosis. *Br J Dis Chest* 1986;80:360–9.
7 Kearon C, Viviani GR, Killian KJ. Factors influencing work capacity in adolescent idiopathic thoracic scoliosis. *Am Rev Respir Dis* 1993;148:295–303.
8 Menardo-Mazeran G, Michel FB, Menardo JL. Childhood asthma and sports in school: A survey of teachers of sports and physical education. *Rev Mal Respir* 1990;7:45–9.
9 Meyer R, Kroner-Herwig B, Sporkel H. The effects of exercise and induced expectations on visceral perception in asthmatic patients. *J Psychosom Res* 1990; 34:455–60.
10 Clark CJ. The role of physical training in asthma. In: Casaburi R, Petty TL (eds), *Principles and practice of pulmonary rehabilitation.* Philadelphia: WB Saunders, 1993:424–37.
11 Ludwick SK, Jones JW, Jones TK, Fukuhara JT, Strunk RC. Normalization of cardiopulmonary endurance in severely asthmatic children after bicycle ergometry therapy. *J Pediatr* 1986;109:446–51.
12 Strunk RC, Rubin D, Kelly L, *et al.* Determination of fitness in children with asthma: use of standardized tests for functional endurance, body fat composition, flexibility and abdominal strength. *Am J Dis Child* 1988;142:940–4.
13 Cochrane LM, Clark CJ. Benefits and problems of a physical training programme for asthmatic patients. *Thorax* 1990;45:345–51.
14 Freeman W, Stableforth DE, Cayton RM, Morgan MDL. Endurance exercise capacity in adults with cystic fibrosis. *Respir Med* 1993;87:541–9.
15 Orenstein DM, Noyes BE. Cystic fibrosis. In: Casaburi R, Petty TL (eds), *Principles and practice of pulmonary rehabilitation.* Philadelphia: WB Saunders, 1993:439–58.
16 Cerny FJ, Cropp GJ, Bye MR. Hospital therapy improves exercise tolerance and lung function in cystic fibrosis. *Am J Dis Child* 1984;138:261–5.
17 Marcotte JE, Canny GJ, Grisdale R, *et al.* Effects of nutritional status on exercise performance in advanced cystic fibrosis. *Chest* 1986;90:375–9.
18 Orenstein D, Nixon P, Ross E, Kaplan R. Quality of well-being in cystic fibrosis. *Chest* 1989;95:344–7.
19 Fournier M, Derenne J-Ph. Exercise performance in lung transplant recipients. *Eur Respir Rev* 1995;5:38–41.
20 Biggar DG, Feldman Malen J, Trulock EP, Cooper JD. Pulmonary rehabilitation before and after lung transplantation. In: Casaburi R, Petty TL. *Principles and practice of pulmonary rehabilitation.* Philadelphia: WB Saunders, 1993:459–67.
21 Lonsdorfer J, Lampert E, Mettauer B, *et al.* Exercise hyperventilation and fatigue in heart transplants. *Eur Respir Rev* 1995;5(25):18–23.

22 Casaburi R, Patessio A, Ioli F, Zanaboni S, Donner CF, Wasserman K. Reduction in exercise lactic acidosis and ventilation as a result of exercise training in obstructive lung disease. *Am Rev Respir Dis* 1991;**143**:9–18.

23 Burdon JGW, Killian KJ, Jones NL. Pattern of breathing during exercise in patients with interstitial lung disease. *Thorax* 1983;**38**:778–84.

24 Miller A, Brown LK, Sloane MF, Bhuptani A, Teirstein AS. Cardiorespiratory responses to incremental exercise in sarcoidosis patients with normal spirometry. *Chest* 1995;**107**:323–9.

25 DiRocco PJ, Vaccaro P. Cardiopulmonary functioning in adolescent patients with mild idiopathic scoliosis. *Arch Phys Med Rehabil* 1988;**69**:198–201.

26 Kesten S, Garfinkel SK, Wright T, Rebuck AS. Impaired exercise capacity in adults with moderate scoliosis. *Chest* 1991;**99**:663–6.

27 Shneerson JM. The cardiorespiratory response to exercise in thoracic scoliosis. *Thorax* 1978;**33**:457–63.

28 Shneerson JM. Pulmonary artery pressure in thoracic scoliosis during and after exercise while breathing air and pure oxygen. *Thorax* 1978;**33**:747–54.

29 Lyager S, Naeraa N, Pedersen OF. Cardiopulmonary response to exercise in patients with neuromuscular disease. *Respiration* 1984;**45**:89–99.

30 Shepherd RJ. Sports medicine and the wheelchair athlete. In: Wood SC, Roach RC (eds), *Sports and exercise medicine*. New York: Marcel Dekker, Inc, 1994: 41–62.

31 Foster S, Thomas HM. Pulmonary rehabilitation in lung disease other than chronic obstructive pulmonary disease. *Am Rev Respir Dis* 1990;**141**:601–4.

32 Orenstein DM, Reed ME, Grogan FT, Crawford LV. Exercise conditioning in children with asthma. *J Pediatr* 1985;**106**:556–60.

33 Nickerson BG, Bautista DB, Namey MA, Richards W, Keens TG. Distance running improves fitness in asthmatic children without pulmonary complications or changes in exercise-induced bronchospasm. *Pediatrics* 1983;**71**:147.

34 Orenstein DM, Franklin BA, Doershuk CF, *et al*. Exercise conditioning and cardiopulmonary fitness in cystic fibrosis: the effects of a three month supervised running programme. *Chest* 1981;**80**:392–8.

35 Braggion C, Cornacchia M, Miano A, *et al*. Exercise tolerance and effects of training in young patients with cystic fibrosis and mild airway obstruction. *Paediatr Pulmonol* 1989;**7**:145–52.

36 Zach M, Purrer B, Oberwaldner B. Effect of swimming on forced expiration and sputum clearance in cystic fibrosis. *Lancet* 1981;**ii**:1201–3.

37 Edlund LD, French RW, Herbst JJ, *et al*. Effects of a swimming program on children with cystic fibrosis. *Am J Dis Child* 1986;**140**:80–3.

38 Webb AK, Dodd ME. Exercise and training in adults with cystic fibrosis. In: Hodson M, Geedes D (eds), *Cystic fibrosis*. London: Chapman & Hall, 1995: 397–409.

39 Holzer FJ, Schnall R, Landau LI. The effect of a home exercise programme in children with cystic fibrosis and asthma. *Aust Paediatr J* 1984;**20**:297–301.

40 Wijkstra PJ, TenVergert EM, van Altena R, *et al*. Long term benefits of rehabilitation in the home on quality of life and exercise tolerance in patients with chronic obstructive pulmonary disease. *Thorax* 1995;**50**:824–8.

41 Keens TG, Krastins IRB, Wannamaker EM, *et al*. Ventilatory muscle endurance training in normal subjects and patients with cystic fibrosis. *Am Rev Respir Dis* 1977;**116**:853–60.

42 Asher MI, Pardy RL, Coates AL, *et al*. The effects of inspiratory muscle training in patients with cystic fibrosis. *Am Rev Respir Dis* 1982;**126**:855–9.

43 Mier A, Redington A, Brophy C, Hodson M, Green M. Respiratory muscle function in cystic fibrosis. *Thorax* 1990;**45**:750–2.

44 Strauss GD, Osher A, Wang C, *et al*. Variable weight training in cystic fibrosis. *Chest* 1992;**92**:273–6.

45 Novitch RS, Thomas HM. Rehabilitation of patients with chronic ventilatory limitation from nonobstructive lung disease. In: Casaburi R, Petty TL (eds), *Principles and practice of pulmonary rehabilitation*. Philadelphia: WB Saunders, 1993:416–23.

46 Novitch RS, Thomas HM. Pulmonary rehabilitation in patients with interstitial lung disease. *Am J Respir Crit Care Med* 1995;**151**:A684.

47 Johnson EW, Braddom R. Over-work weakness in facioscapulohumeral muscular dystrophy. *Arch Phys Med Rehabil* 1971;**52**:333–6.

48 Gross D, Ladd HW, Riley EJ, Macklem PT, Grassino A. The effect of training on strength and endurance of the diaphragm in quadriplegia. *Am J Med* 1980; **68**:27–35.

49 Estrup C, Lyager S, Noeraa N, Olsen C. Effect of respiratory muscle training in patients with neuromuscular diseases and in normals. *Respiration* 1986;**50**: 36–43.

50 Simonds AK, Parker RA, Branthwaite MA. The effect of intermittent positive-pressure hyperinflation in restrictive chest wall disease. *Respiration* 1989;**55**: 136–43.

51 Wanke T, Toifl K, Merkle M, Formanek D, Lahrmann H, Zwick H. Inspiratory muscle training in patients with Duchenne muscular dystrophy. *Chest* 1994; **105**:475–82.

52 Bar-Or O, Blimkie CJR, Hay JA, *et al*. Voluntary dehydration and heat intolerance in cystic fibrosis. *Lancet* 1992;**339**:696–9.

53 Smith K, Cook D, Guyatt GH, Madhavan J, Oxman AD. Respiratory muscle training in chronic airflow limitation: a meta-analysis. *Am Rev Respir Dis* 1992; **145**:533–9.

54 Sassi-Dambron DE, Eakin EG, Ries AL, Kaplan RM. Treatment of dyspnea in COPD. A controlled clinical trial of dyspnea management strategies. *Chest* 1995;**107**:724–9.

55 Fisher AP. NIH Workshop Summary. Pulmonary rehabilitation research. *Am J Respir Crit Care Med* 1994;**149**:825–33.

56 Ambrosino N, Capodaglio P, Bazzini G, *et al*. Simulation of daily activities as functional rehabilitation in COPD patients. *Am J Respir Crit Care Med* 1995; **151**:A683.

12 Travel for technology dependent patients with respiratory disease

F SMEETS

Before becoming disabled by lung disease most patients have lived a normal family, social, and professional life. While the disease progresses slowly the patient manages a "normal life" characterised by the slower pace of daily activities, the material constraints of medical treatment, the precautions necessary to cope with transportation, the practical need to rearrange living space, and the ever present signs of the disease—namely cough, expectoration, and dyspnoea on minimal physical exertion.[1]

Once patients become dependent on oxygen their lives change dramatically. The tubing links them to their oxygen source and symbolises the end of independence and the fulfilling of interpersonal relations. Travelling under such conditions seems completely unthinkable, primarily because of the technical difficulties involved. Nevertheless, people with a respiratory handicap are still capable of travelling, providing they receive the necessary encouragement and advice.

Active participation in a pulmonary rehabilitation programme can enable patients to gradually regain self confidence, merge their equipment with daily life, and improve their physical condition.[2] In 1985 Burns[3] initiated a Caribbean cruise for oxygen dependent respiratory patients and, since 1986, Belgium's "Association des Insuffisants Respiratoires" (AIR) has organised 20 medically supervised trips to various international destinations for more than 500 patients with chronic obstructive pulmonary disease (COPD), including some 30 oxygen dependent individuals.[4] Their mean forced expiratory volume in one second (FEV_1) was one litre, with one third of the patients having a value between 500 ml and one litre.

236

Car travel

Providing adequate oxygen to a patient who is travelling by car will depend on the type of oxygen source the patient is using at home, the number of hours of oxygen required, and the length of the stay away from home. The situation is quite different in patients receiving continuous oxygen from those having oxygen only at night. If the patient is on a concentrator 24 hours a day he or she is very unlikely to undertake travel. If, however, oxygen is required at night only—that is, 15 hours a day, it is practical to take the oxygen concentrator along and to plug it in wherever the patient stays (remembering international voltage differences).

So called "portable" concentrators can be plugged into the car battery, thereby enabling oxygen to be administered while travelling. Unfortunately portable concentrators have a very limited ability (one or two hours of oxygen) and the commercial distribution network is still rudimentary in Europe. Although pressurised oxygen cylinders are no longer used for long term oxygen therapy, they may prove useful for travel. Small 400 litre cylinders will provide 2–3 hours of oxygen at a flow rate of 2 l/min, and 1000 litre cylinders, which are normally easy to transport by car, provide eight hours supply. It is also perfectly feasible to use an oxygen concentrator at night and cylinders during the car journey, providing the patient is not dependent on oxygen for 24 hours a day and can walk without oxygen.

In theory, liquid oxygen is the only form of oxygen that truly frees the patient to move about, given the 7–8 hour supply contained in the portable reservoirs. Beyond this timespan the patient must return to the oxygen source to "fill up" the portable system. If the patient is away from the liquid source for more than 7–8 hours an "economiser" nasal device can be used to increase the period of autonomy by some 40%.

Transporting liquid oxygen tanks by car is possible but the tank must be either tightly strapped to the back seat or, preferably, carried in the boot (trunk) of the car. A smaller tank is available that will fit more easily into the boot. A wooden frame should be used to immobilise the tank in the boot. Given the steady evaporation of the oxygen, the boot must be well ventilated by fitting an escape vent to allow the oxygen to escape. If the tank is placed in the passenger area, one window should be open to prevent a build up of oxygen.

Air travel

Today, flying is accessible to almost everyone. It has been estimated that 5% of commercial airline passengers have some disease or illness including COPD.[5] Furthermore, a growing number of patients on long term oxygen therapy (LTOT) are now flying. This raises special problems because of the hypoxaemia associated with high altitude flying.

The main American carriers take 8–12 oxygen dependent passengers on their flights weekly.[6] In Europe SAS carry 500–600 passengers each year who require inflight oxygen. Iberian Airways carried 120 passengers who required oxygen in 1991, and Swissair supplied oxygen to 129 passengers in the last six months of 1992. Aer Lingus estimates the number of oxygen dependent passengers on its flights to be 70–80 a year, and KLM quote the same order of magnitude (84 patients in 1991). Lufthansa carried 151 oxygen dependent passengers in 1991, Finnair said it had had only a handful of oxygen dependent passengers over the past year, and Sabena provides supplementary oxygen at least three times a week (between 150 and 200 passengers per year).

Physiological considerations

Aircraft usually fly at altitudes of up to 12 500 metres (41 000 feet). All commercial airliners are pressurised so that the cabin pressure is higher than the outside atmospheric pressure.[7] Most of the time the cabin is kept at a pressure equivalent to that at 1600–2500 metres (5000–8000 feet) above sea level (Table 12.1).

International aviation regulations recommend that aircraft flying at their maximum authorised altitudes should keep the cabin pressure equal to that at 2438 metres or 8000 feet.[8] At a cabin pressure equivalent to the atmospheric pressure at 2500 metres the partial oxygen pressure (Pao_2) of a normal, healthy passenger will drop to 8·6–9 kPa (65–68 mm Hg),[9] which still lies on the horizontal part of the oxyhaemoglobin dissociation curve, and saturation will drop 3–4%. In contrast, significant hypoxaemia and desaturation may develop in patients with chronic lung disease[10–12] as they often start with an ambient Pao_2 near to the end of the horizontal part of the oxygen dissociation curve.

Although firm data are scanty, medical aid was required for one in every 100 000 passengers (one in 1900 flights) on one American carrier, and 10% of these cases were for a respiratory disorder.

Table 12.1   Differential pressures and cabin altitudes of different commercial aircraft at a flight altitude of 35 000 feet (10 700 metres)

Aircraft	Differential pressure* (psi)	Cabin altitude in feet (metres)
B-727	8·6	5400 (1646)
B-737	7·45	8000 (2438)
B-757	8·6	5400 (1646)
B-767	8·6	5400 (1646)
B-747	8·9	4700 (1433)
DC-8	8·77	5000 (1524)
DC-9	7·76	7300 (2225)
DC-10	8·6	5400 (1646)
A-300	8·25	6100 (1859)
A-320	8·3	6000 (1829)
L-1011	8·4	5800 (1768)
BAC-111	7·5	7900 (2408)
Concorde	10·7	1000 (305)

*Pressure differential between cabin and outside air as a result of aircraft compression in pounds per square inch (psi). (Modified from Gong.[21])

The global inflight death rate was one per 6400 000 passengers between 1976 and 1979.[13] Later statistics covering the period from 1977 to 1984 give an inflight mortality rate of 0·31 per million passengers, with respiratory ailments accounting for only 6% of the total number of deaths.[14]

According to studies on the use of long term domiciliary oxygen,[15 16] oxygen therapy should be administered to patients with COPD who have PaO_2 levels below 55 mm Hg when they fly at cabin pressures corresponding to altitudes of 1600–2200 metres (5000–7000 feet).[17] Many studies, however, indicate that stable COPD patients may remain asymptomatic and withstand brief altitude induced hypoxaemia (PaO_2 30–40 mm Hg or 4–5·3 kPa) relatively well, even without supplementary oxygen.[17–20] Most of the patients studied were normocapnic rather than hypercapnic and did not have any coexisting cardiac disease. Although the incidence of inflight exacerbations of pulmonary disease seems relatively low, the number of incidents in at risk passengers that might have been avoided by preventive administration of oxygen is not known.[21]

Nomograms and various equations have been developed to estimate a patient's PaO_2 value during a flight. Gong et al[18] developed a formula that uses two variables—the ground PaO_2 value and the altitude in feet—which is valid for altitudes from 1500 to 3000 metres (5000 to 10 000 feet) (Figure 12.1).

239

Oxygen at altitude and on aircraft

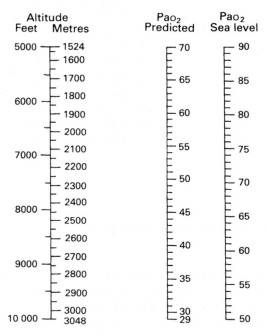

Figure 12.1 Nomogram for predicting altitude Pao_2 (5000–10 000 feet) in normocapnic patients with COPD ar sea level. A straight line connecting sea level Pao_2 and the anticipated altitude will intersect the predicted altitude Pao_2. The lower 95% confidence limits range between 0·6 and 1·8 mm Hg below the predicted altitude Pao_2 throughout the designated ranges of sea level Pao_2 and altitude. (Reprinted with permission from Gong.[21])

Gong *et al*[18] have also developed a high altitude hypoxia simulation test (HAST) in which the potential passenger breathes a hypoxic mixture of gases corresponding to the altitude at which he will be flying. This enables the amount of oxygen that the patient will require during the flight to maintain an adequate Pao_2 to be determined, as well as the cardiovascular and neuropsychological changes that the hypoxia may induce and the efficacy of supplemental oxygen. This test is particularly useful in the case of patients who are already hypercapnic.

240

In practice the Pao_2 measured on the ground remains the most reliable value for predicting the Pao_2 at high altitudes and thus an inability to withstand altitude.[17 18 22-24] If the preflight Pao_2 is less than 70 mm Hg (9·3 kPa) provision must be made for supplemental oxygen to be available, as the maximum Pao_2 drop at 2500 metres (8000 feet) is of the order of 30–35 mm Hg (4·0–4·7 kPa) in all pulmonary patients, even in pressurised cabins.[25] Gong[26] thus recommends prescribing inflight oxygen for all patients whose Pao_2 level may drop below 50 mm Hg (6·7 kPa).

Despite the considerable arterial hypoxaemia at moderate altitudes in these patients, its clinical consequences are still uncertain.[26-28]

Practical considerations for the patients

The request

A request for inflight continuous oxygen during the entire flight must be submitted to the airline's medical department using the INCAD form (standard for all 120 affiliates of the International Air Transport Association) at least 48 hours before departure. This form is provided by the travel agent and must accompany the reservation. The form, filled in by the physician, includes information about the patient's itinerary, flights, specific medical data (diagnosis, prognosis, treatment, clinical state), and the oxygen needs: flow rate and amount of oxygen required. In estimating the oxygen needs one must allow for the flying altitude and possible take-off and landing delays. Adding 60 minutes would be a reasonable safety margin. The patient should always have a copy of his medical form available.

As there are no specific guidelines for inflight oxygen therapy,[29] each airline company has its own regulations. Some companies limit the number of oxygen dependent passengers they will take on the same flight.[6] In addition, airlines are not obliged to take passengers requiring continuous oxygen.

It is of vital importance to check on the day before the departure that the necessary steps have been taken to ensure that a sufficient amount of oxygen will be available during the flight.[6] Patients should follow up on all arrangements to be sure that their needs are understood by everyone.

Cabin service

Although the medical departments of airlines are generally familiar with the problem of oxygen dependent passengers, the flight attendants usually have only limited knowledge. They sometimes tend to seat such passengers at the back of the cabin in the smoking area! One must insist firmly on a seat in the forward, non-smoking section of the cabin, preferably an aisle seat near the toilets.

In no case may the patient use his own oxygen equipment on board.[30] Portable reservoirs may be brought along empty, either as hand luggage or checked baggage. If the tank is taken along it, too, must be empty. Liquid oxygen is not allowed on aircraft.[31][32]

Airline companies will usually supply oxygen cylinders which are strapped beneath the passenger's seat. Although the large 3000 litre cylinders usually have metered valves allowing variable flow from 2 to 8 l/min, the small 300 litre cylinders have fixed flow rates of either 2 or 4 l/min.

The airline companies usually supply facemasks instead of nasal prongs. These masks are rather uncomfortable, especially when they have to be worn for several hours. Patients should take their own prongs with them, as well as tubing. There may be some problems fitting them to the oxygen bottles of the aircraft: a good pair of scissors, a pocket knife, and some extra connectors may be useful.

Ground service at the airport

Airline companies cannot provide oxygen for ground use before boarding, after landing, and at any stopovers. If the patient can do without oxygen while checking in and boarding, there is no problem. For those who are totally dependent on oxygen it may be necessary to use the patient's own portable reservoir during boarding operations until entering the plane, at which point the security staff must take the equipment and return it to the check in desk where a member of the patient's family can recover it.

If there are stopovers where the patient must get off or change flights, it will be necessary to prearrange (usually through the oxygen distributor) for someone to meet the flight with supplementary oxygen.

Cost of inflight oxygen therapy

Most airline companies charge a supplemental for providing inflight oxygen that can range from $US40 to $US200 per flight.

The service is usually billed for each flight rather than for the litres of oxygen actually used, which is why direct flights are preferable to connecting flights.

General recommendations

The patient must take on board all the medication that is likely to be needed during the flight, especially metered dose aerosols. A battery powered ultrasonic nebuliser may be useful during the flight. These are permitted providing they do not disturb the other passengers and no electrical interference with the plane's communications circuits is possible.[33]

During the flight the patient should avoid overeating and drinking alcoholic beverages; it is important to keep well hydrated because of the relative dryness of the cabin air: the usual temperature is 20–22°C, the relative humidity is low (10–12%), and the cabin air is renewed every three minutes.[34]

It is prudent for an oxygen dependent patient to be accompanied when flying by a companion or spouse who will be able to help if needed.

Cruises

The coastguard regulations regarding transport of liquid oxygen even for medical use are very strict. Most shipping companies, however, allow oxygen dependent patients to travel with either their oxygen concentrators or a tank of liquid oxygen. When booking the patient must notify them of the permanent need for oxygen and each company will have to refer the matter to its own medical department, which will require a medical report specifying the diagnosis and oxygen needs.[35 36]

Cruises are particularly suitable for respiratory patients because there are no problems of altitude, pollen, or pollution likely to trigger bronchial spasms.

Travel for patients on mechanical ventilators

There are currently an estimated 8000 patients worldwide using mechanical ventilators at home, a quarter of whom require treatment 24 hours a day.[37]

France and the United States of America have the most experience in this area. The National Center for Home Mechanical

Ventilation in the United States of America has enrolled over 350 patients to date (B Make, personal communication), and ANTADIR in France[38] monitors 2000 patients on mechanical ventilation.

The most frequent indications for their use are neuromuscular disorders, kyphoscoliosis, sometimes COPD, and sleep apnoea. The most frequently used equipment in Europe is the Monnal-D respirator. Patients are connected to the respirator by a tracheostomy or, more often, a noseclip or facemask. Some of these patients are also oxygen dependent.

One might assume that only patients who make intermittent use of mechanical ventilation are likely to travel. Only patients with kyphoscoliosis and sleep apnoea syndromes and COPD, however, enjoy enough autonomy to be able to consider travelling when stabilised.

There is no information available on the number of patients receiving ventilation who travel. Their number will probably increase as more continuous positive airway pressure (CPAP) and BiPAP systems are prescribed to treat sleep apnoea. Nevertheless, night ventilation remains a cumbersome treatment that the patient already finds difficult to accept at home. Travelling with this equipment will require much energy and courage.

Eurolung Assistance is a network for respiratory patients in Europe and has been in operation for five years. The 1991/92 directory[39] lists not only medical departments directly involved in pulmonary rehabilitation and oxygen therapy, but also medical equipment and oxygen suppliers. The main oxygen distributors have their own international and worldwide distribution network and can supply the oxygen needs to a patient at the intended destination as long as they are active in that location. France has, in addition, a network of home care associations (ANTADIR) that patients can use when they travel.

Some travel companies and associations offer professionally supervised travel opportunities for people with respiratory insufficiency requiring 24 hour oxygen. In Europe the recent association of Wagons-Lits Travel, Vitalaire, the insurance company l'Européenne, and the Association des Insuffisants Respiratoires has made it possible to handle all arrangements needed by these patients. "Life Unlimited" in Florida offers the same service.

When travelling abroad a special travel insurance is mandatory. In case of a road accident the insurance company will take charge of all the costs of the repatriation. In case a sudden unexpected disease is diagnosed, the hospital costs will also be covered. But what about an acute exacerbation of the underlying COPD? Often the condition of travel insurance will not cover any "pre-existing" disease, so a hospital stay for an acute exacerbation during the holiday may not be covered by the insurance. It is therefore very important for the patient to specify any pre-existing chronic pulmonary disease, particularly oxygen dependent patients who are at greater risk. Not all insurance companies will cover this supplementary risk.

Conclusions

Travelling remains possible for individuals with respiratory handicaps, even for those who are severely limited by the need for constant oxygen therapy, provided certain precautions are taken:

1 Pulmonary rehabilitation: participating in such a programme enables the patient to learn more about the illness and thus cope with it and manage it better. Respiratory re-education and physical retraining improve the patient's physical condition. A patient should go on vacation only if "stable" and feeling reasonably well.
2 Strict planning: a trip for an oxygen dependent person cannot be improvised. It must be prepared well in advance. This includes choosing the location, time of year, climate, means of transportation, travelling companion, and taking steps to ensure the continuation of medical treatment, medical resources on site, and oxygen supplies. Taking part in a group trip with medical supervision specially designed for patients with COPD might be a good start.
3 Think ahead: nothing should be left to chance during the trip. The maximum number of difficulties that may crop up should be foreseen and planned for.

The time when the COPD patient's world stopped at the end of the 15 metre tubing that bound him to his oxygen concentrator is a thing of the past. The world is now within reach of the oxygen dependent person. If the physician can convince the patient to try at least one trip to an unfamiliar destination he or she may well want to travel again and again.

Appendix

Further information, guidelines, and practical advice regarding travel by patients with pulmonary disease are available from the following sources.

Eurolung Assistance
(F Smeets)
Centre Hospitalier Ste Ode,
6680 Ste Ode, Belgium.
Tel: +32 84 22 52 82.
Fax: +32 84 22 52 84.

Mary Burns,
Little Company of Mary
Hospital,
Torrance, Boulevard 4101,
Torrance, CA 90503, USA.
Tel: +1 213 540 7676.
Fax: +1 213 540 8408.

The Society for the
Advancement of Travel for the
Handicapped
347 Fifth Avenue, Suite 610,
New York, NY 10016, USA.
Tel: +1 212 447 7284.
Fax: +1 212 725 8253.

The Royal Association for
Disability and Rehabilitation
(RADAR)
25 Mortimer Street,
London W1N 8AB, UK.
Tel: +44 71 637 5400.
Fax: +44 71 637 1827.

International Air Transport
Association
2000 Peel Street,
Montreal, Quebec,
Canada H3A 2R4.

Life Unlimited
Robbins, Associates Health
Care Travel Consultants,
1701 SW 200th Street, Z-28,
Miami, Florida 33187, USA.
Tel: +1 305 441 6819.

Association des Insuffisants
Respiratoires (AIR)
56 rue de la Concorde,
1050 Bruxelles, Belgium.
Tel: +32 2 512 29 36.
Fax: +32 2 512 32 73.

Vitalaire
10 rue Cognac-Jay
75341 Paris, Cédex 07,
France.
Tel: +33 1 44 11 00 00.
Fax: +33 1 44 11 00 90.

National Oxygen Travel
Service (NOTS)
2892 South Dixie Drive,
Dayton, Ohio 45409, USA.
Tel: +1 513 297 7397.
Fax: +1 513 297 7396.

G Weinmann AG
Riond Bosson 13,
1110 Morges, Switzerland.
Tel: +41 21 803 5026.
Fax: +41 21 803 5028.

ANTADIR
Boulevard Saint-Michel 66,
75006 Paris, France.
Tel: +33 1 46 33 02 40.
Fax: +33 1 46 33 74 59.

1 Pretet S, Pignier D, Thomas V. *Comment vivre avec un handicapé respiratoires?* Paris: J Lyon, 1992.

2 Donner CF, Howard P. Pulmonary rehabilitation in chronic obstructive pulmonary disease (COPD) with recommendations for its use. *Eur Respir J* 1992;5:266–75.

3 Burns M. Cruising with COPD. *Am J Nurs* 1987;87:479–82.

4 Smeets F. Social life organization for severely disabled respiratory patients. In: *Second International Conference on Advances in Pulmonary Rehabilitation and management of chronic respiratory failure, Venice 1992.* New York: Raven Press, 1993.

5 Iglesias R, Cortes MDCG, Almanza C. Facing air passengers' medical problems while on board. *Aerospace Med* 1974;45:204–6.

6 Gong H Jr. Oxygen at altitude and on aircraft. In: Tiep BL (ed), *Portable oxygen therapy: including oxygen conserving methodology.* Mount Kisco, New York: Futura, 1994.

7 McFarland RA. Human factors in relationship to the development of pressurized cabin. *Aerospace Med* 1971;42:1303–18.

8 Code of Federal Regulations. Title 14, part 25.841. Washington: US Government Printing Office, 1986.

9 Cardiovascular committee of the cystic fibrosis foundation. Airline travel for children with chronic pulmonary disease. *Pediatrics* 1976;57:408–10.

10 Henry JN, Krenis LF, Cutting RT. Hypoxemia during aeromedical evaluation. *Surg Gynecol Obstet* 1973;136:49–53.

11 Air travel for chronic bronchitis. *Lancet* 1984;ii:792–3.

12 Cottrell JJ. Altitude exposures during aircraft flight flying higher. *Chest* 1988;92:81–4.

13 AMA Commission on Emergency Medical Services. Medical aspects of transportation aboard commercial aircraft. *JAMA* 1982;247:1007–11.

14 Cummins RO, Chapman PJC, Chamberlain DA, *et al.* Inflight deaths during commercial air travel. How big is the problem? *JAMA* 1988;259:1983–8.

15 Nocturnal Oxygen Therapy Trial Group. Continuous or nocturnal oxygen therapy in hypoxemia chronic obstructive lung disease. *Ann Intern Med* 1980;93:391–8.

16 Medical Research Council Working Party. Long-term domiciliary oxygen therapy in chronic cor pulmonale complicating chronic bronchitis and emphysema. *Lancet* 1981;i:681–5.

17 Schwartz JS, Bencowitz HZ, Moser KM. Air travel hypoxemia with chronic obstructive pulmonary disease. *Ann Intern Med* 1984;100:473–7.

18 Gong H Jr, Tashkin DP, Lee YE, Simmons MS. Hypoxia altitude stimulation test (HAST): evaluation of patients with chronic airway obstruction (abstract). *Am Rev Respir Dis* 1983;127:86.

19 Graham WGB, Houston CS. Short-term adaptation to moderate altitude: patients with chronic obstructive pulmonary disease. *JAMA* 1978;240:1491–4.

20 Tomashefski JF, Shillito FH, Billings CE, Ashe WF. Effects of moderate altitude on patients with pulmonary and cardiac impairment. *Calif Med* 1964;101:358–62.

21 Gong H Jr. Air travel and oxygen therapy in cardiopulmonary patients. *Chest* 1992;101:1104–13.

22 Dillard TA, Berg BW, Rajagopal KR, Dooley JW, Mehm WJ. Hypoxemia during air travel in patients with chronic obstructive pulmonary disease. *Ann Intern Med* 1989;111:362–7.

23 Bjorkman BA, Selecky PA. High-altitude simulation at rest and exercise to determine oxygen therapy needs in hypoxemia patients during airplane travel: a community hospital experience (abstract). *Chest* 1988;94(suppl):315.

24 Mathur PN, Dowdeswell IRG, Stonehill RB. A method to assess and prescribe controlled oxygen therapy during commercial air travel. *Am Rev Respir Dis* 1984;129(part 2):A51.

25 California Thoracic Society. *Airplane travel information for physicians.* Oakland, California: American Lung Association of California, 1983.

26 Gong H Jr. Air travel and patients with chronic obstructive pulmonary disease (Editorial). *Ann Intern Med* 1984;**100**:595–7.

27 Shillito FH, Tomashefski JF, Ashe WF. The exposure of ambulatory patients to moderate altitudes. *Aerospace Med* 1963;**34**:850–7.

28 Richards PR. The effects of air travel on passengers with cardiovascular and respiratory diseases. *Practitioner* 1973;**210**:232–41.

29 Hong H Jr. Advising pulmonary patients about commercial air travel. *J Respir Dis* 1990;**11**:484–99.

30 Federal Aviation Regulation. Part 121.574. Oxygen for medical use by passengers. Oklahoma City: Federal Aviation Administration.

31 Dangerous Goods Board Committee, International Air Transport Association (IATA). Provisions for dangerous goods carried by passengers or crews. In: *Dangerous goods regulations.* Montreal: IATA, 1990:I:1.7.2(B)3.

32 Council of International Civil Aviation Organization (ICAO). Provisions for dangerous goods carried by passengers or crews. In: *Technical instructions for sage transportation of dangerous goods by air.* Montreal: ICAO, 1989/90:I:2.4.2.C.

33 Poundstone W. Air travel and supplemental oxygen: friendly skies for respiratory patients? *Respir Ther* 1983;**136**:79–82.

24 *International Air Transport Association Medical Manual.* Montreal: International Air Transport Association, 1986.

35 Santoro K. A vacation cruise for COPD patients. *Respir Ther* 1985;**15**:31–5.

36 Olenik PC. Planning a cruise? Know the facts about oxygen transport and use. *AARC Times* 1988;**12**:24–9.

37 Howard P. Home respiratory care. *Eur Respir Rev* 1992;**1**:563–8.

38 Muir J-F. Home mechanical ventilation in patients with chronic obstructive pulmonary disease. *Eur Respir Rev* 1991;**1**:550–62.

39 Smeets F. Eurolung Assistance Directory. *Eur Respir J* 1991;**4**(suppl 14):562S.

13 How to keep the customer satisfied

TREVOR CLAY
Revised by John Isitt

I wear two different hats—one as a health professional and one as a consumer. I spent 35 years in the health care business, in the nursing service, nursing management and, for the last 10 years, at the Royal College of Nursing—in the real politik! I retired on health grounds in 1989—it's strange how we say "health" when we mean "ill health". It seems to have become politically correct. Have you noticed that psychiatric units have become mental health units? Political correctness is hitting health in a big way now, though it doesn't make the problems go away. The fact is that I have probably learned more about some of the vital aspects of health care in the past four years than I did in the previous 35. It is true what they say—there is nothing like first hand experience.

We all remember patients who inspired us and whom we admired. They usually feature early in our careers. A child; someone who dies in great pain; the many, many people who showed great courage and bravery. I personally remember a man called Alfie Lomas. I expect he was in the second half of his fifties and, of course, I thought he was old! He had emphysema and had to struggle to breathe nearly all the time. But he was the sort of chap who made the doctors and nurses (and patients) feel better. He explained to newcomers the ward rules—the need to keep the beds tidy and to lie in bed at attention. He explained the vital importance of the consultant's round, and also that, important though it was, the Matron's round was even more important!

Editor's note: Trevor Clay died in 1994.

249

I learned a lot from Alfie Lomas, but I remember thinking what a gap there was between the quality of his life and mine. I was in that young age group where I thought there would be a cure for death before it got to be my turn. I played tennis and sprung about like Zebedee of "Magic Roundabout" fame, but nevertheless I'd always been a chesty kid and somehow *knew* even then, deep down, that emphysema was to be important in my life.

I want to have a look at how things have changed, and perhaps how they haven't, since Alfie's time. Some specialties have changed beyond recognition in 40 years, but many long term lung conditions haven't changed all that much, or rather, the quality of life of the people with them hasn't. When Alfie was in his early to mid-fifties the NHS was not yet 10 years old and patients were mightily grateful for it. If they ever made the slightest squeak of a complaint it was invariably about something inanimate—like the old red waterproofs they used to have to lie on, or the food. They would say: "The doctors and nurses were wonderful but the food was terrible." That has changed somewhat over the years but is changing even more rapidly now. I hope health professionals will feel able to welcome the new consumerism. It is not, in my view, based on negative views of treatment and care and those who provide it, but is simply of a different time and a society which wants, wherever possible, an equal partnership in the scheme of things. Already one hears less of "Whatever you say doctor" and more of "Let me just see what I'd written on my list, to make sure I've discussed everything I need to". In any case, difficult though it may be to accept, the solution to many of *your* problems may lie in the new consumerism.

The British Lung Foundation, in the United Kingdom, exists to raise money for research into lung disease. I'm proud that its Council and Executive Committee so readily agreed to the setting up of a consumer arm and voice in the shape of Breathe Easy. We now have nearly 10 000 members of the club and my aim is to achieve 100 000 by the end of this century. What has surprised many is the fact that Breathe Easy people want to raise money for lung research just as much as all the fit young people who generously ride bicycles for us. Breathe Easy members are making an increasing contribution to our income.

They also write to us telling us what life is like for them and how they think it could be improved, with lots of constructive suggestions and ideas. From these we have developed an agenda and it is mainly this list of issues which, as we address them

250

and make progress with them, will help to keep the customer satisfied. The main items on the agenda are air pollution; smoking and the guilt often felt by smokers about having done it, as well as the agony of watching people smoking now; the frequent lack of support in the life struggle; the provision of liquid oxygen, or rather the lack of provision, which impedes mobility outside the home; the problem with getting nebulisers (and I mean where they are prescribed); 'flu and whether they should be immunised against it; and social issues such as the availability of incapacity benefit and worries about the imposed VAT on fuel bills (at 8·5%). These issues are matched by hundreds of letters full of positive, helpful advice about how to improve quality of life—from breathing exercises and yoga to the value of blowing up balloons, and—yes—alternative or complementary therapies.

I want to pick out just one issue from this list: that of the lack of support. Huge numbers have written and included phrases like "the doctor told me there is nothing that can be done". That phrase is used to people over and over again. One of my preoccupations is the language we all use and one of my ambitions is to dissuade health professionals from saying "there's nothing more that can be done". Apart from the devastating effect it has on people, it is simply not true. What is meant is that there is no cure, no magic, *but there is always something that can be done.* This isn't just political correctness, but goes to the core of what we need to be addressing.

As we move towards the end of this century and into the next and people live to be older, this situation will be increasingly highlighted. Symptom relief, palliative care, and different health care partnerships have to be high on the agenda for all of us, whichever hats we wear. Just to go back to language for a moment, you'll notice I've committed perhaps the most cardinal sin—I've been talking about people with lung disease, not patients. Of course I'm a patient when I'm with my doctor or when I'm ill, but most of the time I'm not a patient suffering from lung disease but a person living with it. When we're fighting battles for more resources or working together to raise money for this specialty we're doing it for people. Believe me, it is about living. People seem to be as terrified of dying as ever. But having a long term condition is not about dying—that only takes a few minutes or less—but I've been struggling to breathe for over 20 years and I've been living a lot and suffering as little as possible. It is true, though, that you have to have significant resources and in some ways be very strong to cope with any long term condition.

Another area of support in which we are becoming interested is that of peer group support. My own profession has recently set up a Respiratory Nurses Group within the RCN and I'm delighted about this; they have even set up a Nurses Against Smoking Group and I hope that particular charity begins at home—nurses still have one of the worst records, as an occupational group, in failing to give up smoking. But the big thing in respiratory nursing now is "patient education". Nurses, of course, have a significant contribution to make in assisting and supporting people and patients, but I would prefer it if they enabled and facilitated peer groups to help themselves. Breathe Easy now has 39 local groups. In any case, this might be a better use of professional nursing time.

The answer to the question of how to keep the customers satisfied is therefore fairly simple—we need to get closer to each other, the health professionals and the customers, and to share more with each other. My plea is to let the customers in. We need to unite on issues like smoking (and the progress the libertarian lobby has been making while we haven't been looking) and, above all, to press for more research into preventing lung disease and improving the lives of people who have it now. To do that we need to raise the public profile of the lung even more than has been managed so far. Society needs to know that we are united and passionate about all these issues.

These are troubled times for many in the health service. Recently the Audit Commission issued yet another of its reports about the health service. I get as riled as you must to see a body like this telling us what's what. I am bound to say, though, that I get even more riled at the fact that they're usually right. This latest missive is about information and is entitled "Listen more to patients". Health professionals are besieged from all sides with pressures as well as advice. It's a new world in health care in this country. Alfie would not recognise it. I'm not sure Bevan or Beveridge would either! NHS Trusts are nothing if not challenging (I serve as a non-executive member of a Trust Board) and in many parts of the United Kingdom 1994/95 means doing more work for no more or even less money in many specialties—where does all that extra money politicians keep talking about go to?

If health professionals are experiencing low morale and having to fight harder than ever for their specialty, then part of the solution lies in a strong partnership with consumers. In all the areas where real progress and a higher profile have been achieved it has been done in this way, often, indeed, led by the consumers.

Our concern is about the very air we breathe into some of the most delicate and sensitive organs in the body. Maybe our turn has come; the issues are relevant and important and timely enough. Let's breathe new life into getting change and improvements for people with lung disease—and those who care about them.

Index

255

transdiaphragmatic pressure
(Pdi) 46–7
treadmill test 196–8
treadmill walking 103

V slope criterion 25
Vential (SAIME) 153, 155(fig)
Ventil + (SEFAM) 153, 155(fig)
ventilators 151–3

volume cycled, available in
Europe 154(fig)
ventilatory muscle training 45–63
methods 52–5
outstanding issues 60–2
rationale 51–2
response 55–60
Vitalaire 244, 246

walking test 103–4, 196